DEDICATION

I want to dedicate this book to my wife, Laura (my biggest fitness fan, supporter and proofreader), family, fitness clients, friends, and mostly to the people that always ask me health and fitness questions anywhere I go, or through all my social networks. Thanks to them, I was inspired to put these workouts together, along with the healthy eating tips, and share my knowledge and passion for health and fitness.

Special thanks to Tracy McCutchion for her graphic design work, to Cynthia Westendick for her fitness modeling contribution, and to Glen Dykstra, Bryan Spear, and Kym Trice for their photography.

Copyright © 2013 The Trainer, LLC

This work is copyright protected. The unauthorized reproduction of all or portions of this book, in any form whatsoever, is prohibited, without written permission from the author.

31 DAYS OF FAT BURNING WORKOUTS

INTRODUCTION

Hello, my name is Marcelo Vazquez. I am a fitness professional and the creator of Spin-Fit™ (www.spin-fit.com). Every day I get health and fitness questions about what to eat, what kinds of workouts are best for strengthening the core, burning more calories, getting leaner arms, stronger legs, sexy shoulders, or a flat stomach. So, I decided to create workouts based on these health and fitness questions and to make them available to you. If your goal is to lose weight, or get leaner and stronger, then this book is for you. These 31-days of fat burning workouts, the healthy eating tips, the motivational quotes of the day, and the video tutorials will give you the confidence and determination to start a fitness program and keep going until you get your desired results.

Why 31 days? It is very easy to create bad habits and very hard to break them. It takes about 21 days for the body to start developing any new habit, so I did not want to stop in the middle of the month. I decided to go for the entire month worth of workouts. Here is an example of how new habits start developing in your body. If you set the alarm at 6am every day, after 3 weeks, you will probably wake up by yourself before the alarm goes off. If you try to drink coffee or tea without sugar, the beginning will be rough, but in a few weeks your body will adapt to this new taste, and it will not miss the sugar. Just try! I will help you stick to 31 days of working out. Your body will adapt to a new fitness habit, and as you keep going, your body will get stronger and it will crave more and longer workouts (more rounds).

These 31-days of fat burning workouts consist of five exercises per round, combining high and low intensity exercises to burn calories and fat. Ideally you go from one to five rounds per workout. If you are a beginner, I will not expect you to start doing five rounds per workout every day beginning day one. Try to do one to two rounds per day, and then keep increasing the rounds. The rounds can be done during the day in bouts of five minutes without having to do them all at once. Please do not punish yourself trying to get faster results, if you do that, more than getting faster results, you may quit, because it is insane and you might get injured. Besides, I want you to get into the habit of working out every day as part of your lifestyle, rather than a short-term fitness goal. So, start slow with 1-2 rounds at a time; after 31 days, your body will adapt to this new way of life and next month, you will go for an extra round. Just listen to your body, your body will tell you when it is ready to move to the next level.

Now, make up your mind and pledge that no matter what, you are going to stick with these 31-days of fat burning workouts, from Day 1 to Day 31. Your body is a masterpiece and it is capable of doing many things that you are not aware of, so keep a positive mental attitude in every workout. Soon you will realize that you are stronger than you think, and nothing will stop you from conquering your fitness goals. Besides, you can count on me, Trainer Marcelo, to answer any questions you might have through my different social networks. So, what are you waiting for, small decisions make big differences. Get ready to begin your journey towards a new YOU! I will be there to motivate and encourage you, and remember your progress is our SUCCESS. Let's begin!

Marcelo Vazquez

ATTENTION

Please consult your physician before starting this or any other fitness program. All material provided in this workout is for informational and educational purposes only. You agree that use of this information is at your own risk and hold THE TRAINER LLC, the instructor(s), the crew, facility or any persons involved with this event, testing procedure or video production, harmless of any responsibility from any and all losses, liabilities, injuries or damages resulting from any and all claims.

If at any point of your workout you begin to feel dizzy, faint or have any physical discomfort, STOP immediately and consult your physician. You are responsible for exercising within your limits and seeking medical advice and attention as appropriate. A 5-10 minute warm-up walk or jog, and a 5-10 minute cool-down of stretching are recommended. A mat is suggested for floor exercises.

31 DAYS OF FAT BURNING WORKOUTS

SOME OF THE HEALTH BENEFITS OF BEING ACTIVE

Here are some of the many health benefits of being active.

- **Strengthening the Heart:** the more you exercise the stronger your heart becomes. A stronger heart will pump more blood through the body with less effort. A fit person will also have a lower heart rate at rest, compared to someone that is unfit. A healthy and strong heart will increase the chances of living longer.

- **Weight Control:** it is easy to gain weight and it is very challenging to lose. You gain weight when the calories you eat and drink are greater than the calories you burn. Healthy eating and physical activity play a critical role in controlling your weight.

- **Strengthening Bones and Muscles:** aging is inevitable, and after 30, you start losing bone density and muscle strength. That is why it is very important to minimize this loss by planning for and performing a daily exercise routine.

- **Reducing the Risk of Cardiovascular Disease:** even 30 minutes a day of brisk walking can help minimize the risk of cardiovascular disease. You can reduce this risk further by adding more physical activity to your day. Increasing your physical activity can also minimize blood pressure and improve good cholesterol levels.

- **Reducing the Risk of Type 2 Diabetes:** insulin helps the cells to absorb the blood sugar that is used as fuel. Even short periods of exercise can improve the sensitivity of muscles to insulin.

31 DAYS OF FAT BURNING WORKOUTS

- **Improving Mood:** daily exercise can reduce the risk of stress, anxiety, and depression. It may also help you to sleep better and improve self-esteem.
- **Improving Sex Life:** daily exercise will make you look good and feel more energetic, creating a positive effect on your sex life. Also, men that exercise regularly are less likely to have erectile dysfunction problems than those that don't exercise.

MIND AND BODY CONNECTION

Start this program by training your mind over your body. Because I do not want you to stop or skip workouts, make up your mind that nothing will stop you from accomplishing your fitness goals. Start slow, take periodic breaks between rounds if needed. Little by little your body will adapt to the training and will ask you for more. It is very important that you keep a positive mental attitude every day to keep the connection going.

Stress is one of the factors that can disrupt your connection between mind and body, so you have to identify and be aware of the factors that interfere with your connection. Your body responds to the way you think and feel. If you feel stressed, your body will tell you that something is not right. Some signs of stress are:

- Low back pain
- Shoulder tightness
- Neck ache
- Headache
- Chest pain
- Erectile dysfunction

- Insomnia
- Heart palpitations
- Weight gain or loss

Once you recognize these signals, try to minimize the level of stress to recover your connection between mind and body. Try to talk about these stress factors with family and friends to find ways to minimize stress. Remember, minor discomfort is different than pain. If these signs of stress persist, continue to work with your physician to determine the causes and how your exercise routines may need to be modified to allow you to exercise safely.

Even if you have stress under control, you might find yourself disconnected from your workout. For instance, if you are working out and your mind is somewhere else, you will not have the same results as if your mind is concentrated on the muscle you are working. When you recognize this disconnection, PUSH yourself anyway and at least do one round to get back on track. A shorter workout is better than no workout at all. Besides, you will feel much happier. Why? Because when you exercise, your brain releases chemical substances called endorphins. Endorphins are responsible for changing your emotional state and can make you feel happy. So, keep pushing for a happier you!

MOTIVATION – THE 10 BEST WAYS TO KEEP YOU GOING

Motivation is easy to acquire and hard to maintain. When you feel fired up, GO, and do as much as you can. Do as many rounds as you possibly can, but remember, work within your limits. Go the extra mile because some days you will find yourself unmotivated and you will not do as many

31 DAYS OF FAT BURNING WORKOUTS

rounds as you do when you are fired up. Remember that everything starts in your mind; PUSH and your body will follow. Here are a few ideas to keep the motivation up:

1. Just do your workout, **don't think** about it. Push yourself to do the first round of your workout and you will get into the mood. Many times you may not feel like working out, but once you start, the adrenaline runs through your body and soon your emotional state changes. Sometimes the mind betrays the body by convincing the body it is too tired to exercise. Think for a moment, if you have been sitting at a desk all day long, you probably ARE mentally tired, but your body is fresh and ready to exercise. As soon as you get back from work, and before you hit the couch, put your tennis shoes on and go for a walk, jog or run.

2. Turn unproductive time into workout time by **planning** in advance. For example, if you know you are going to be stuck in traffic for one hour after work, why leave the office? Bring your workout clothes and plan to do a few rounds at the office. Change that wasted time in traffic for some productive workout time. Besides, after you are done with your workout, the traffic will be reduced, and when you arrive home, you can enjoy spending time with family or enjoying your favorite show or game, guilt-free.

3. Put workout items by the door as **reminders** to exercise every time you leave the house. Prepare your workout bag the night before and put it by the door, so you have to run into that bag on your way to work. Buy a cool pair of tennis shoes and put them by the door to motivate you to exercise.

4. Sometimes you may need a **partner** to exercise with, to motivate you. Ideally your partner will be the same gender and have similar fitness goals. Why, because males tend to acquire results faster than females, so if

you are a female working out with your male partner or spouse, he might have results faster than you and this might be discouraging. On the other hand, if you exercise with another female with similar goals, you can exchange fitness ideas and encourage and motivate each other to eat healthy and exercise daily.

5. **Music** can be very motivational as well. Play your favorite music and find "the" song that will make you take the first move and keep going and going. When you need a little push, play "your" song. You can also dance 2-3 songs non-stop as a warm up to get ready to start your first round.

6. A piece of **clothing** can be part of the motivation, too. Find a dress that's too small, a pair of jeans, or a bikini and put this item where you can see it every day, like by the mirror, in the bedroom, or why not next to the refrigerator. The more you see the item, the more you will be determined to exercise and eat clean. You can also try the item on periodically to monitor your progress.

7. Find a **picture** of yourself at your ideal weight. Make sure you put that picture where you can see it every day to keep the motivation flowing. Put that picture by the mirror, in your wallet or at your desk. The more you see it, the closer you will be to achieving your goal.

8. **Fuel up first.** Eat a snack like fruit, low-fat yogurt, or an all-natural health bar before working out. Exercising on an empty stomach might make you feel dizzy and unmotivated to keep going, due to low blood sugar. By fueling up first you will increase your energy level and the motivation to exercise, and eventually you can burn more calories.

9. Step on the **scale** weekly. Weigh yourself every Monday at the same time of the day. Usually people tend to

"behave" with the calories they consume from drinks and foods during the week, and misbehave during the weekend. Thinking about the scale on Monday, you will be motivated to ingest calories in moderation, and exercise to burn them off before Monday.

10. Look for **help within;** you might find it during your workout. In the same way that stress can disrupt the balance between mind and body, when you have something on your mind that is disturbing you, you may not feel motivated to exercise. When you exercise your mind becomes focused and exercise wakes the happy chemicals in your brain called "endorphins". During or after a workout, you may just discover the solution you have been looking for.

I am sure you can find what motivates you to keep going - a health issue, a promise, a New Year's resolution or just to look and feel good. Whatever it is that keeps you motivated, find it and stick with it**.** Your results will come sooner than you think if you keep your motivation up. Feeling happy, work out; feeling down, work out; in doubt, keep working out!

PROPER NUTRITION

Do not forget that for optimal results you have to fuel your body properly. To successfully burn fat you have to eat. Food is energy and to be able to burn fat you have to fuel up first. Skipping meals will slow down your metabolism. So, try to eat small healthy meals every 2-3 hours to keep all the nutrients coming and keep your metabolism going. Here are examples of important nutrients and the roles they play in your body.

Carbohydrates are preferred by the body as the main source of energy. Carbohydrates are stored as glycogen in both the liver and muscles, and liver glycogen is easily converted to energy. There are two kinds of carbohydrates. Simple carbohydrates are usually found in foods with fewer nutrients, and tend to be less satisfying and more fattening. Examples are sugar, corn syrup, candy, baked goods made with white flour, and some packaged cereals. Complex carbohydrates are derived from plants that contain both starch and fiber. Examples are vegetables, potatoes, dried beans, grains and fruits. The bottom line is, minimize the consumption of carbohydrates that are sugary and consume carbohydrates that are high in fiber and nutrients.

Fat is another important nutrient. After carbohydrate stores have been depleted, fat is then metabolized for energy production. Examples of good fat, which your body needs in healthy quantities, are olive oil, avocados, nuts, and fatty fish (salmon, tuna, sardines).

Protein is tapped into when there are times of no food intake over extended periods. In times of carbohydrate restriction or during extreme activity, protein is also used to make glucose for fuel. Protein is responsible for muscle repair, maintenance and growth. Examples are eggs, beans, fish, poultry, and lean meats.

Water is the most important nutrient and accounts for about 70% of overall body mass. It is very important to consume fluids before, during and after working out. Drink plenty of water throughout the day to make sure your body is well hydrated. Do not wait until you are thirsty to drink water; thirst is a symptom of dehydration. Remember, your body will need more water during hot days.

31 DAYS OF FAT BURNING WORKOUTS

This is just a little information about nutrients, and how they play an important role in your workouts and overall performance. It is **a must** to consult a registered dietitian when a meal plan is needed to accompany a workout routine. For training purposes, stay away from (or minimize) foods that are high in calories like sugars, fried foods, white flour (switch to whole grains), and alcohol. Alcohol is high in sugar and does not provide any nutrients.

SUGGESTED FOOD TIMING – 5 MEALS PER DAY

Don't forget that your body needs nutrients to keep your metabolism going. Here is an example of how I fuel my body during the day.

- **Breakfast:** Whole grain cereals, low-fat milk products, and healthy proteins (from eggs and nuts)
- **Middle Morning and Afternoon Snacks:** Fruit of choice, low-fat yogurt, celery and carrot sticks, or dried fruits and nuts
- **Lunch:** Grains, protein, fruits and vegetables in approximately equal parts.
- **Dinner (not after 8:30pm):** Mainly high in protein and low in carbohydrates.
- **Within an Hour after Working Out**: High-protein meal to recover. Use protein shakes as a last resort.

FITNESS LEVEL

Make sure you consult with your physician before starting this or any other fitness program.

31 DAYS OF FAT BURNING WORKOUTS

- **Beginners**: start slow, take your time, and do not rush. Let your body and muscles adapt to a new habit. Later, as you get more comfortable with the exercises, you can gradually increase the rounds. Do at least one round at a time, at your own pace, creating your own exercise routine. Remember, always exercise within your limits.

- **Intermediate**: once your body adapts, it will get stronger and stronger, and it will ask you for more. Then, is the time to increase rounds, and you might be comfortable doing three rounds. Always listen to your body, it will tell you when it is time to go for more. Keep in mind that for best results you should take minimal or no rest between exercises.

- **Advanced**: now that you created a new habit of working out every day, and doing three rounds is not enough, add one more round to complete four, then five. Be patient and keep doing your rounds every day. Soon you will realize that you can add more bouts during the day for best results and faster weight loss. Like the intermediate level, take minimal or no rest between exercises for best results.

The beauty of these workouts is that the only equipment you need is your own body weight, and the workouts can be done anywhere you go. Some exercises are timed and some are by number of repetitions. If you do not like to count you can always use a range of 30-45 seconds per exercise. There is no need to buy an expensive timing device, a stop watch will do the job, or if you have a smart phone, get a free app that will help you with your workouts. My favorite free timer app is by Gymboss Interval Timer. If you do not like to time yourself, you can always transform the seconds in the workout to numbers of repetitions, for instance 30 seconds = 30 repetitions. I like to do both timing and number of

31 DAYS OF FAT BURNING WORKOUTS

repetitions to add variation, avoid boredom and spice up the workout.

HIGH AND LOW INTENSITY FOR BEST RESULTS

As mentioned before, once carbohydrates are depleted, fat will be used as energy. Most people have enough fat stored to keep exercising and burning without running out of fuel. At low intensity you can still burn fat which is why I like to do ab workouts in combination with a few rounds from the **previous 2-3 days of workouts**. The abdominal muscle group is like any other muscle; to strengthen the abs you have to work them. Once you start burning the fat that is covering the abs, eventually, you are going to be able to see the desired six-pack.

To burn fat and build the desired six-pack you need a combination of high and low intensity workouts, and strength training to build lean muscle. The more lean muscle you can build, the more you can burn because muscle has to burn calories to keep functioning.

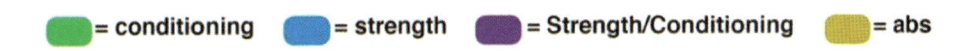

● = conditioning   ● = strength   ● = Strength/Conditioning   ● = abs

Conditioning (Cardio): During cardio exercise, the first nutrients that the body burns are carbohydrates (transformed into glucose). When the body runs out of this fuel source, it will begin using fat as fuel. Throughout the workouts you will find these high intensity exercises indicated in green.

Strength: Working with resistance (like using your own body weight) will help build lean muscle. The more lean muscle you can build, the more you can burn. Throughout

31 DAYS OF FAT BURNING WORKOUTS

the workouts you will find these low intensity exercises indicated in blue.

Strength/Conditioning: Combining conditioning with strength training is a great way to burn calories and fat, and build lean muscle. Throughout the workouts you will find both low and high intensity exercises indicated in purple.

Low impact (abs): my preferred way to strengthen the core, burn fat, and build the desired six-pack. The perfect combination would be to start with 2-3 rounds from previous workout days and then do the regular ab workout of the day. That way you can increase the blood circulation, raise heart rate, feel the burn, and get a great abdominal routine. Throughout the workouts you will find these low intensity exercises indicated in yellow.

These workouts are diverse to keep your body guessing and working harder. If you do the same exercises every day, eventually you are going to get bored, and your muscles will get bored as well. For instance, if you do cardio on the elliptical machine every day, there is going to be a point of time where your muscles will say "again the same exercise?!" and they will become bored, lazy, and burn less fat, even if you feel the sweat running down your face. Create muscle confusion to avoid boredom and keep your muscles guessing, working and burning in every workout.

THE UNWANTED FAT

It takes 3500 calories to gain a pound of fat. If you want to lose a pound per week, reduce your calorie intake by 250 calories per day and incorporate daily physical activity that will burn an additional 250 calories.

Do not get fooled by weight loss programs or products that claim to help you lose weight fast without exercising. Losing weight is one thing, burning fat is another. These programs or products often use restricted diets to lose weight. However, you are just losing WATER and MUSCLE MASS, putting your body at risk, and depriving your body of many nutrients. The fat will still be there, because you did not do anything to burn it off. So when you stop the weight lost program or using the products, you gain more weight.

There is no shortcut, magic potion, or secret. To lose weight and burn fat you have to exercise. Furthermore, there is not a specific exercise that will burn fat in one specific area of the body. When you exercise you burn fat from any spot where there is extra fat like in thighs, buttocks, under arms, or the abdomen area. So, keep doing your daily exercises to get rid of the unwanted fat.

MUSCLE SORENESS

If you are a beginner to exercise, it is normal to get muscle soreness after working out. This soreness is called DOMS (Delayed Onset Muscle Soreness), but do not be alarmed, this soreness or discomfort will go away in 48 hours. This discomfort occurs for different reasons. One reason could be because you never exercise, your muscles were sleeping and untrained. Suddenly you wake them up by working out and your muscles are confused. As your muscle are adapting to the new exercise or workout, these muscle groups will make you aware, through soreness, that they are doing something new.

The second reason could be muscle confusion. When you do an exercise repeatedly (like elliptical training) your muscles build a habit. Then suddenly, when you switch to a different exercise (like weight lifting) you confuse your muscles by doing something new. Again, your muscles will let you know with soreness.

A third reason could be increased resistance. For instance, you are lifting weights and you add more resistance to push a little harder. Your muscles will notice this new resistance or weight addition, and will alert you with temporary soreness. So, if you never exercise, switch to different drills/exercises, or if you increase the resistance/weights, your muscles will get DOMS.

It is very important that you learn the difference between discomfort and pain. If you have a minor discomfort, this means that the muscles are adjusting to your new exercise or workout routine. If the discomfort keeps going and becomes painful, STOP immediately and consult your physician.

SAFETY IS FIRST

Always keep safety in mind while working out. You might be eager to start and neglect some safety issues. If you get hurt you will delay your goal of daily fat burning. Here are some safety reminders:

- Do not wear open-toed shoes working out.
- Wear comfortable clothing.
- Wear tennis shoes with thick soles to absorb the impact against the ground.
- Use a beach towel or a mat to do floor exercises.
- Hydrate by drinking plenty of liquids before, during and after working out.
- Avoid wearing jewelry during your workout.

- Avoid wearing lotions, makeup, or any other chemical on your face. As you perspire the chemicals could run into your eyes and create an irritation forcing you to stop.

GET READY AND LET'S BEGIN

Now that you understand the health benefits of being active, how your mind and body are connected, the importance of fueling your body, muscle confusion, and the difference between losing weight and burning fat, let's begin.

If you are a beginner take your time between exercises. Do not rush, it is better if you take periodic rests than trying to rush and finish with bad posture. The more you practice these workouts, the better you will get, and your muscles will adapt and ask you for more, so listen to your body and keep pushing when it is ready.

Remember, you can always divide your workout into small bouts throughout the day. Let's say that you have time early in the morning, and before you hit the shower, you do 1-3 rounds. During your lunch break, do another 1-3 rounds of the same workout of the day. At night, before you turn on the TV, do the final 1-3 rounds. That way you can complete a great workout without spending too much time at once. The best part is that any of these workouts can be done from the comfort of your own place, office, or hotel room, and without the need for any equipment.

Ok, this is basic information to get you started with your workouts and finish the first 31 days of your new healthy lifestyle. I hope you enjoy my program as much as I enjoyed putting it together for you. Remember that you are not alone in this journey; you can always count on me as your fitness partner in case you have any questions or need a little push

31 DAYS OF FAT BURNING WORKOUTS

to keep going. Just Facebook me and together we will move forward. My greatest personal satisfaction would be to help you get the results you always wanted, so you can become an inspiration for others. Keep a positive mental attitude, and remember that you are stronger than you think. The results are closer than you can imagine!

Happy Fat Burning Workouts!

31 DAYS OF FAT BURNING WORKOUTS

ATTENTION

Please consult your physician before starting this or any other fitness program. All material provided in this workout is for informational and educational purposes only. You agree that use of this information is at your own risk and hold THE TRAINER LLC, the instructor(s), the crew, facility or any persons involved with this event, testing procedure or video production, harmless of any responsibility from any and all losses, liabilities, injuries or damages resulting from any and all claims.

If at any point of your workout you begin to feel dizzy, faint or have any physical discomfort, STOP immediately and consult your physician. You are responsible for exercising within your limits and seeking medical advice and attention as appropriate. A 5-10 minute warm-up walk or jog, and a 5-10 minute cool-down of stretching are recommended. A mat is suggested for floor exercises.

DAY 1

MOTIVATION

Why wait when you can start your workout today.

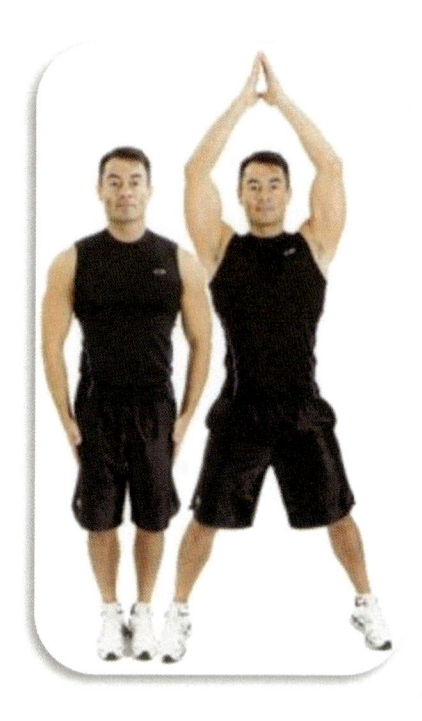

HEALTHY EATING TIP

Read nutrition labels to help you choose foods with little added sugars, fats, and salt.

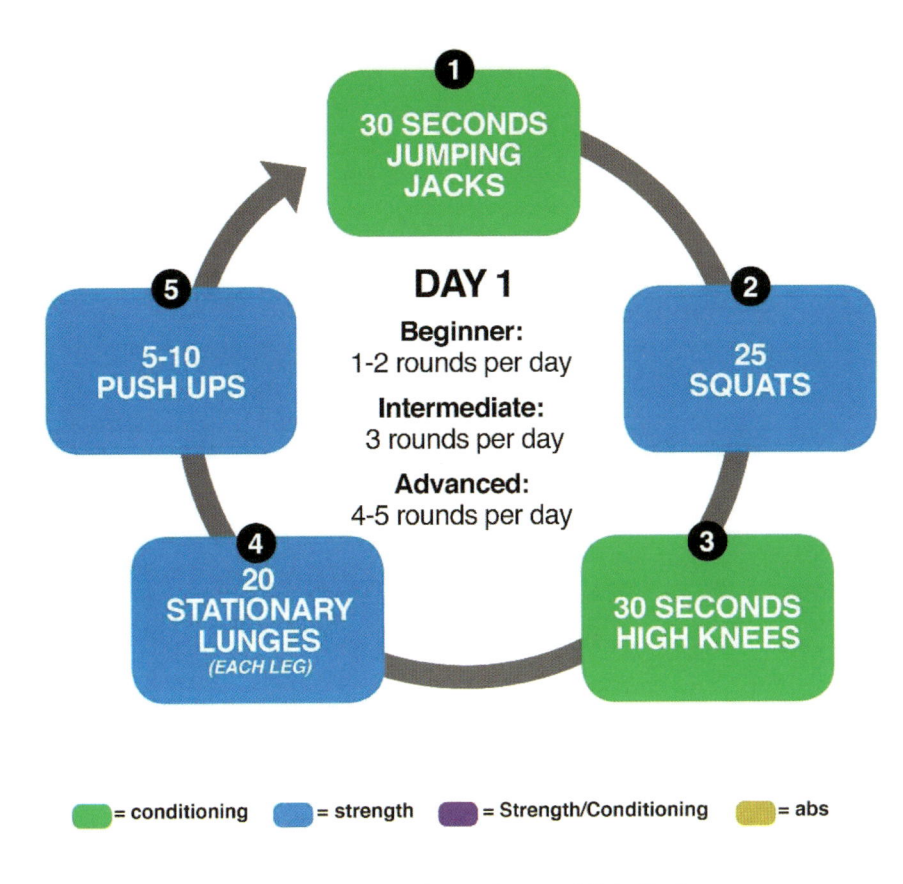

DAY 1

1. 30 SECONDS JUMPING JACKS
2. 25 SQUATS
3. 30 SECONDS HIGH KNEES
4. 20 STATIONARY LUNGES (EACH LEG)
5. 5-10 PUSH UPS

Beginner: 1-2 rounds per day
Intermediate: 3 rounds per day
Advanced: 4-5 rounds per day

- = conditioning
- = strength
- = Strength/Conditioning
- = abs

Warm up prior to workout http://bit.ly/10YPaIU

Bonus Video-Tutorial Day 1 http://bit.ly/13ICGLz

31 DAYS OF FAT BURNING WORKOUTS

DAY 2

MOTIVATION

To achive your goals just give them a try.

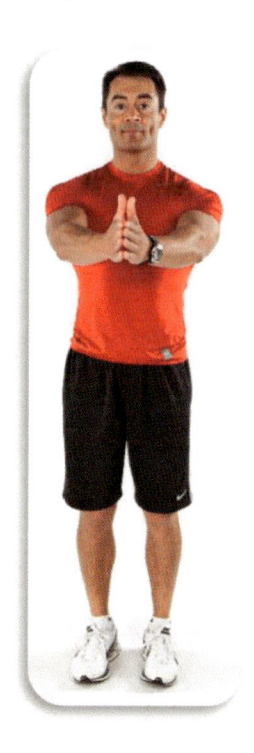

HEALTHY EATING TIP

Eat small meals every 2-3 hours to keep your metabolism working throughout the day.

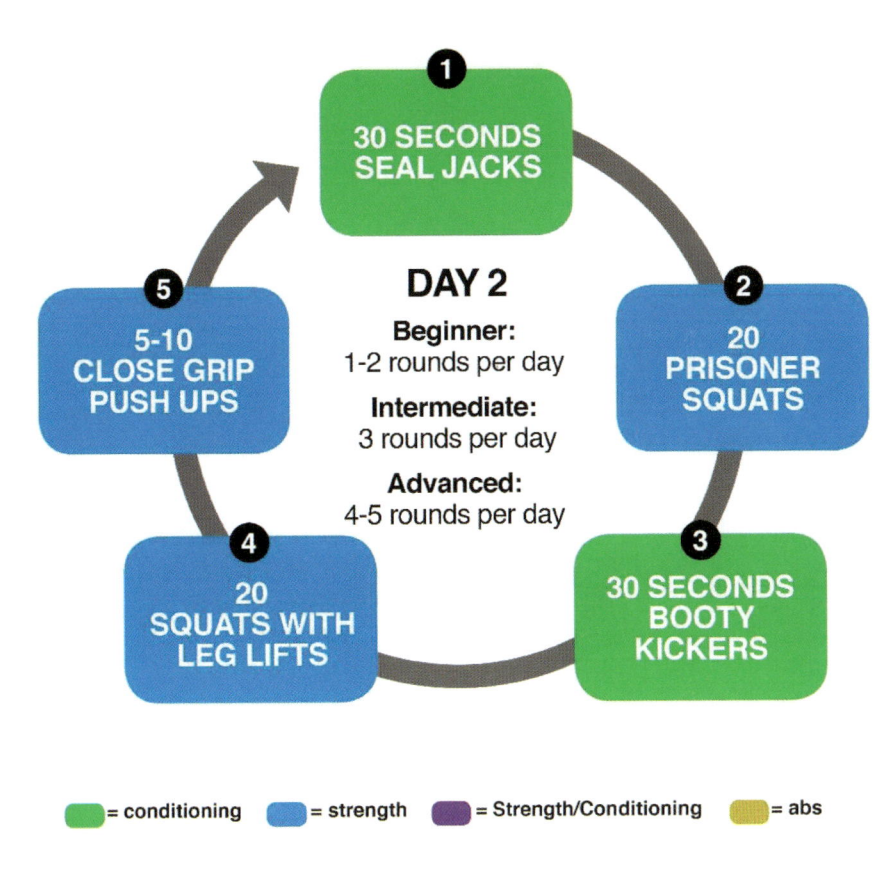

DAY 2

Beginner: 1-2 rounds per day

Intermediate: 3 rounds per day

Advanced: 4-5 rounds per day

1. 30 SECONDS SEAL JACKS
2. 20 PRISONER SQUATS
3. 30 SECONDS BOOTY KICKERS
4. 20 SQUATS WITH LEG LIFTS
5. 5-10 CLOSE GRIP PUSH UPS

🟩 = conditioning 🟦 = strength 🟪 = Strength/Conditioning 🟨 = abs

Warm up prior to workout http://bit.ly/1oYPaIU

Bonus Video-Tutorial Day 2 http://bit.ly/17QEj9t

31 DAYS OF FAT BURNING WORKOUTS

DAY 3

MOTIVATION

Start taking care of yourself and you will inspire others.

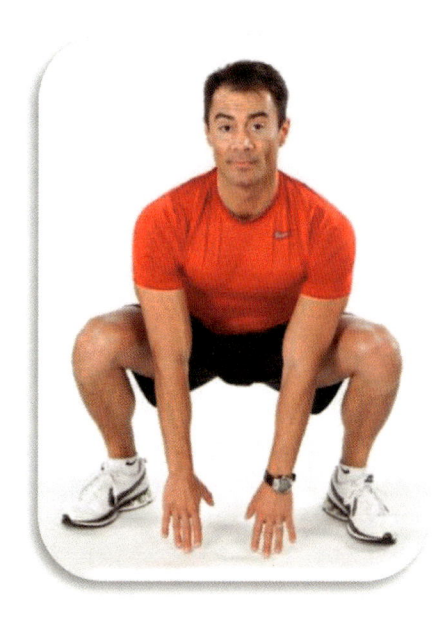

HEALTHY EATING TIP

To lose weight, minimize the consumption of items high in calories like sugar, white flour, fried foods and alcohol.

31 DAYS OF FAT BURNING WORKOUTS

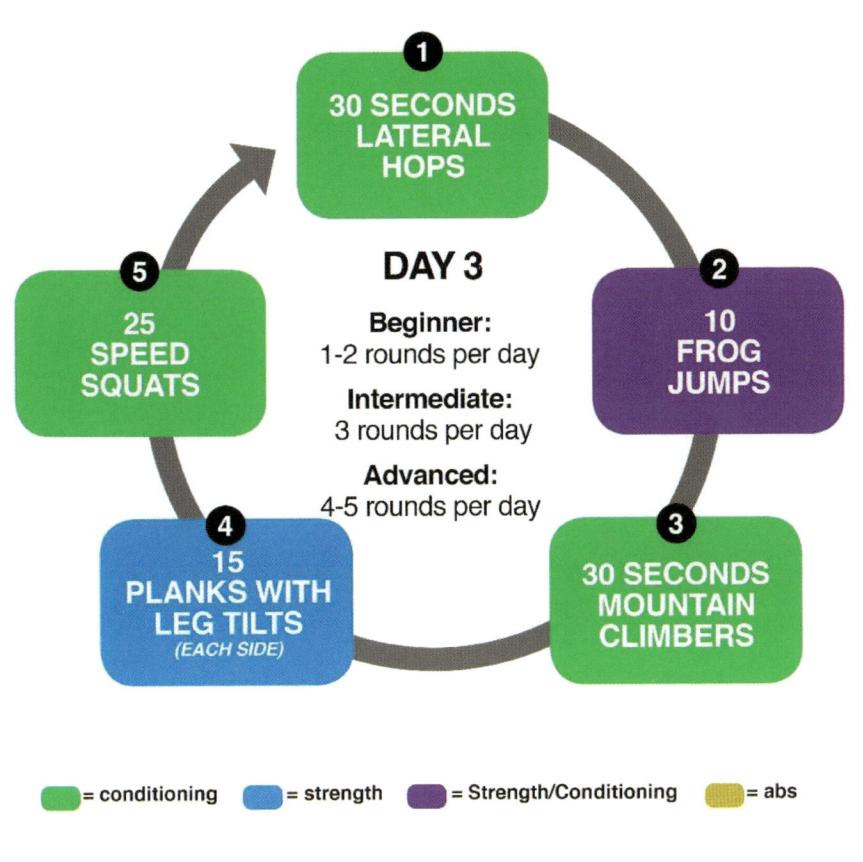

DAY 3

Beginner: 1-2 rounds per day

Intermediate: 3 rounds per day

Advanced: 4-5 rounds per day

1. 30 SECONDS LATERAL HOPS
2. 10 FROG JUMPS
3. 30 SECONDS MOUNTAIN CLIMBERS
4. 15 PLANKS WITH LEG TILTS (EACH SIDE)
5. 25 SPEED SQUATS

- = conditioning
- = strength
- = Strength/Conditioning
- = abs

Warm up prior to workout http://bit.ly/10YPaIU

Bonus Video-Tutorial Day 3 http://bit.ly/17QEtxD

DAY 4

MOTIVATION

Enthusiasm will help you reach your goal.

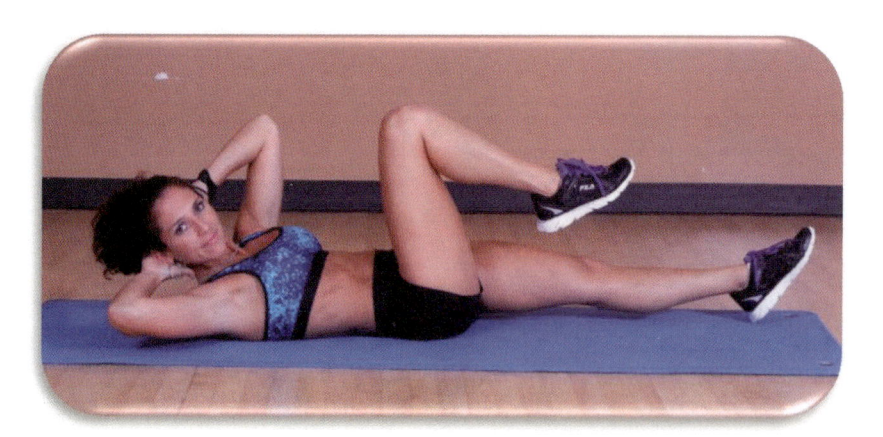

HEALTHY EATING TIP

Drink plenty of water throughout the day to keep your body hydrated. Being dehydrated can make you feel hungry.

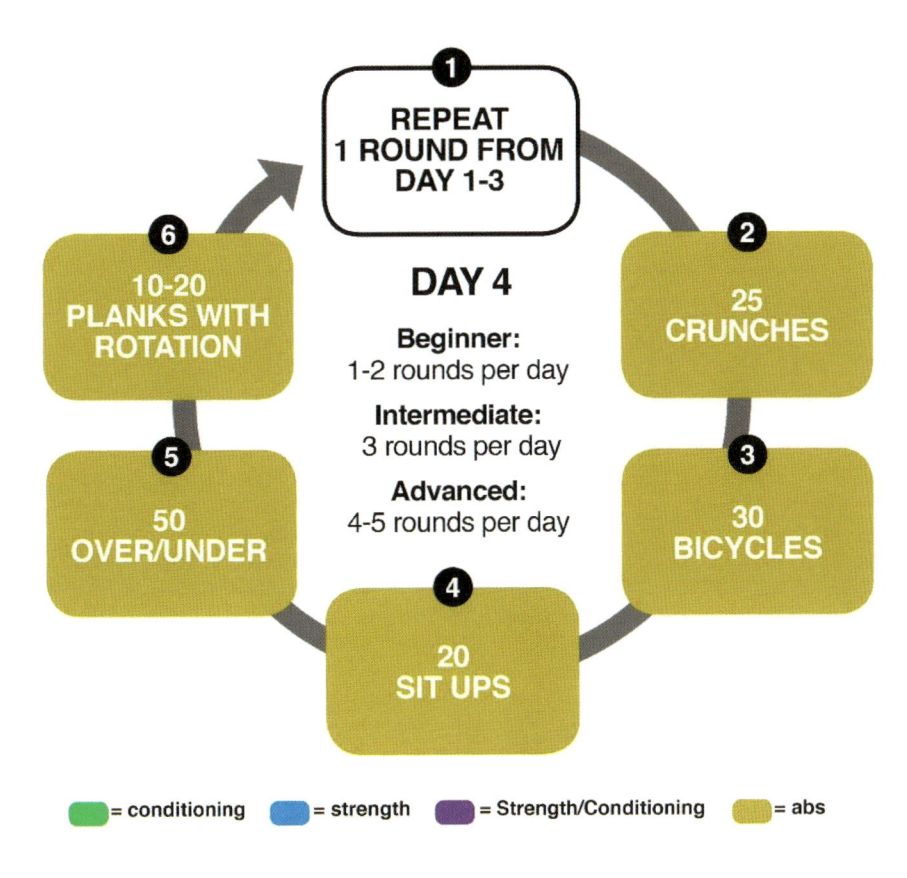

DAY 4

Beginner: 1-2 rounds per day

Intermediate: 3 rounds per day

Advanced: 4-5 rounds per day

1. REPEAT 1 ROUND FROM DAY 1-3
2. 25 CRUNCHES
3. 30 BICYCLES
4. 20 SIT UPS
5. 50 OVER/UNDER
6. 10-20 PLANKS WITH ROTATION

= conditioning   = strength   = Strength/Conditioning   = abs

Warm up prior to workout http://bit.ly/10YPaIU

Bonus Video-Tutorial Day 4 http://bit.ly/15z68DZ

31 DAYS OF FAT BURNING WORKOUTS

DAY 5

MOTIVATION

The power of 3D: be dedicated, be determined, be disciplined.

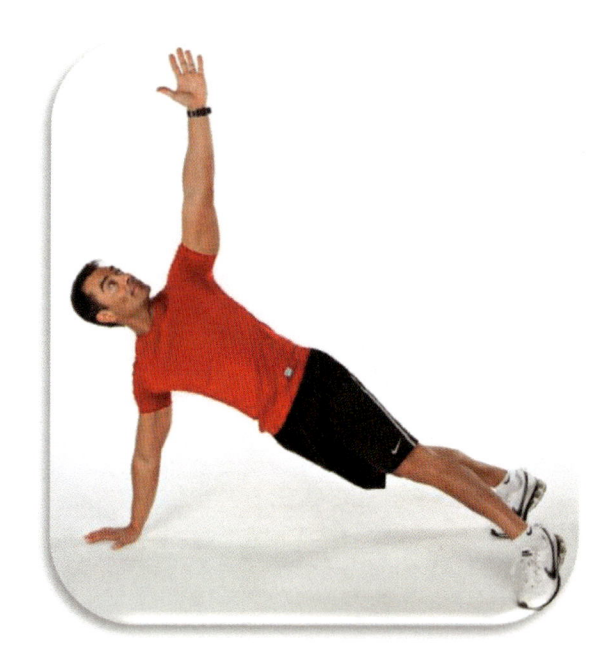

HEALTHY EATING TIP

Store leftovers in single serving containers for portion control and to limit calorie intake.

31 DAYS OF FAT BURNING WORKOUTS

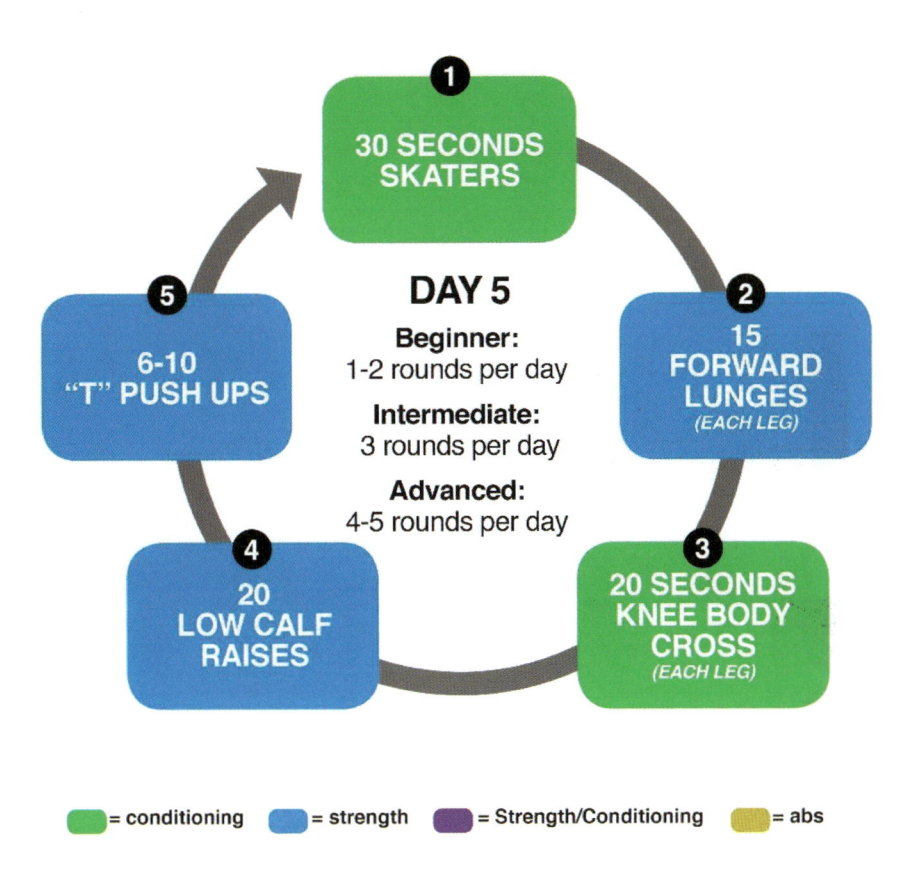

DAY 5

1. 30 SECONDS SKATERS

2. 15 FORWARD LUNGES (EACH LEG)

3. 20 SECONDS KNEE BODY CROSS (EACH LEG)

4. 20 LOW CALF RAISES

5. 6-10 "T" PUSH UPS

Beginner: 1-2 rounds per day
Intermediate: 3 rounds per day
Advanced: 4-5 rounds per day

- = conditioning
- = strength
- = Strength/Conditioning
- = abs

Warm up prior to workout http://bit.ly/10YPaIU

Bonus Video-Tutorial Day 5 http://bit.ly/11uwot

DAY 6

MOTIVATION

You are invincible, unstoppable, and awesome; YES YOU!

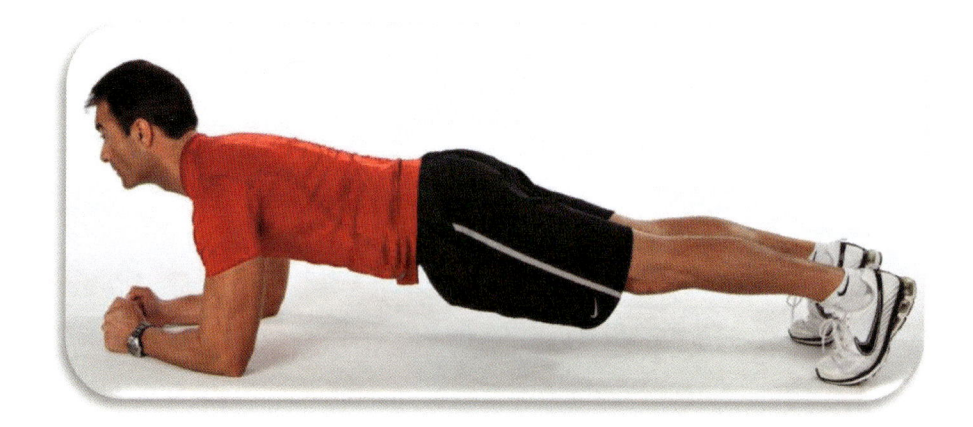

HEALTHY EATING TIP

Be careful with products that are marked as "low-fat", these products are not always the healthiest choice since some manufacturers add more sugar to compensate for the lack of flavor from reduced fat.

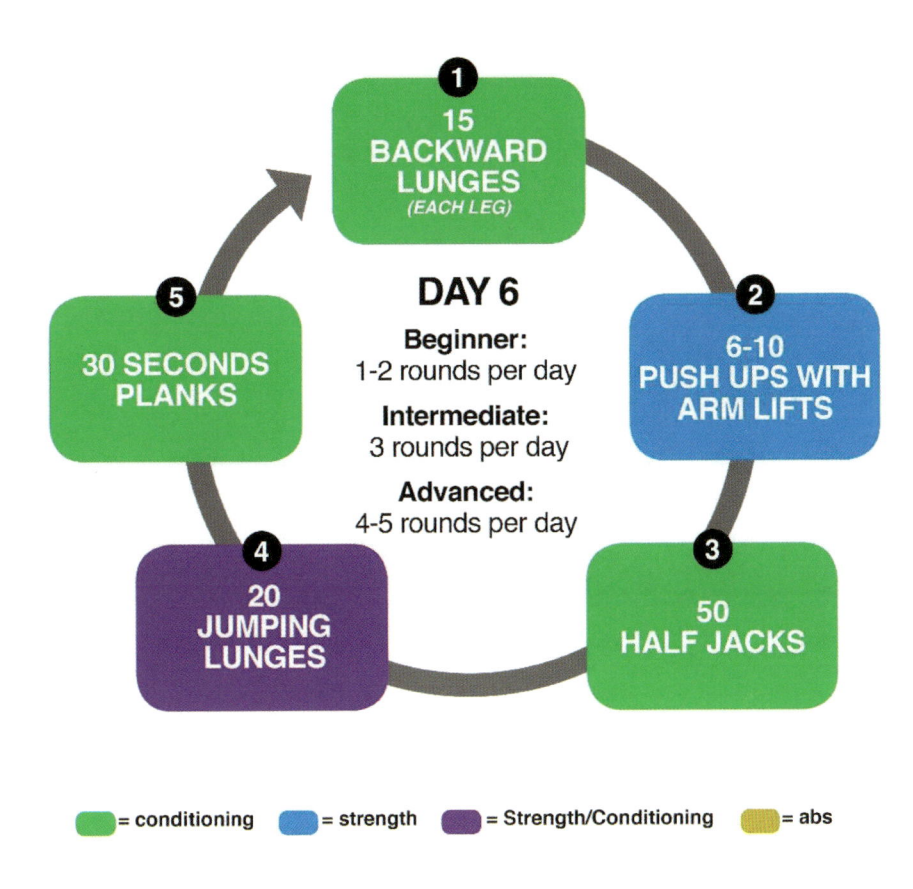

DAY 6

Beginner: 1-2 rounds per day

Intermediate: 3 rounds per day

Advanced: 4-5 rounds per day

1. 15 BACKWARD LUNGES (EACH LEG)
2. 6-10 PUSH UPS WITH ARM LIFTS
3. 50 HALF JACKS
4. 20 JUMPING LUNGES
5. 30 SECONDS PLANKS

🟩 = conditioning 🟦 = strength 🟪 = Strength/Conditioning 🟨 = abs

Warm up prior to workout http://bit.ly/10YPaIU

Bonus Video-Tutorial Day 6 http://bit.ly/Zez4of

- 31 -

31 DAYS OF FAT BURNING WORKOUTS

DAY 7

MOTIVATION

If it's too easy, it doesn't count; always challenge yourself.

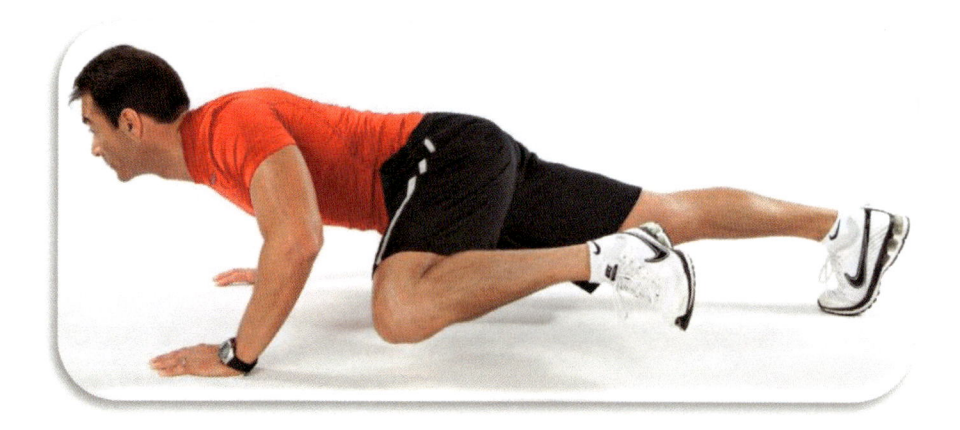

HEALTHY EATING TIP

Combine healthy food choices with an active lifestyle to prevent weight gain.

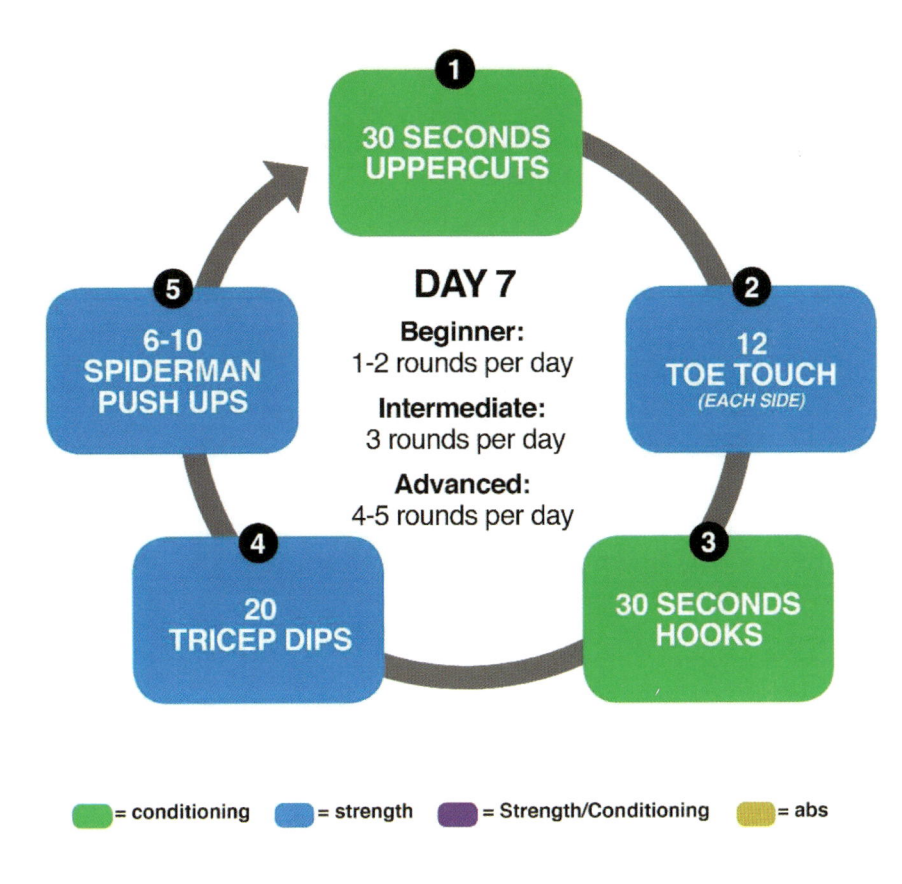

DAY 7

1. 30 SECONDS UPPERCUTS

2. 12 TOE TOUCH *(EACH SIDE)*

3. 30 SECONDS HOOKS

4. 20 TRICEP DIPS

5. 6-10 SPIDERMAN PUSH UPS

Beginner: 1-2 rounds per day

Intermediate: 3 rounds per day

Advanced: 4-5 rounds per day

- 🟩 = conditioning
- 🟦 = strength
- 🟪 = Strength/Conditioning
- 🟨 = abs

Warm up prior to workout http://bit.ly/10YPaIU

Bonus Video-Tutorial Day 7 http://bit.ly/11wrHiT

31 DAYS OF FAT BURNING WORKOUTS

DAY 8

MOTIVATION

Every day that passes will never come back again; enjoy it to the fullest, stay positive and work out.

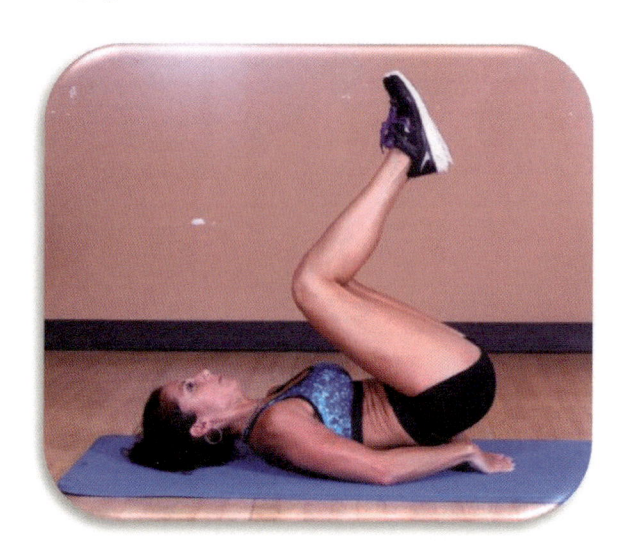

HEALTHY EATING TIP

Serve food on smaller plates to limit calorie intake.

31 DAYS OF FAT BURNING WORKOUTS

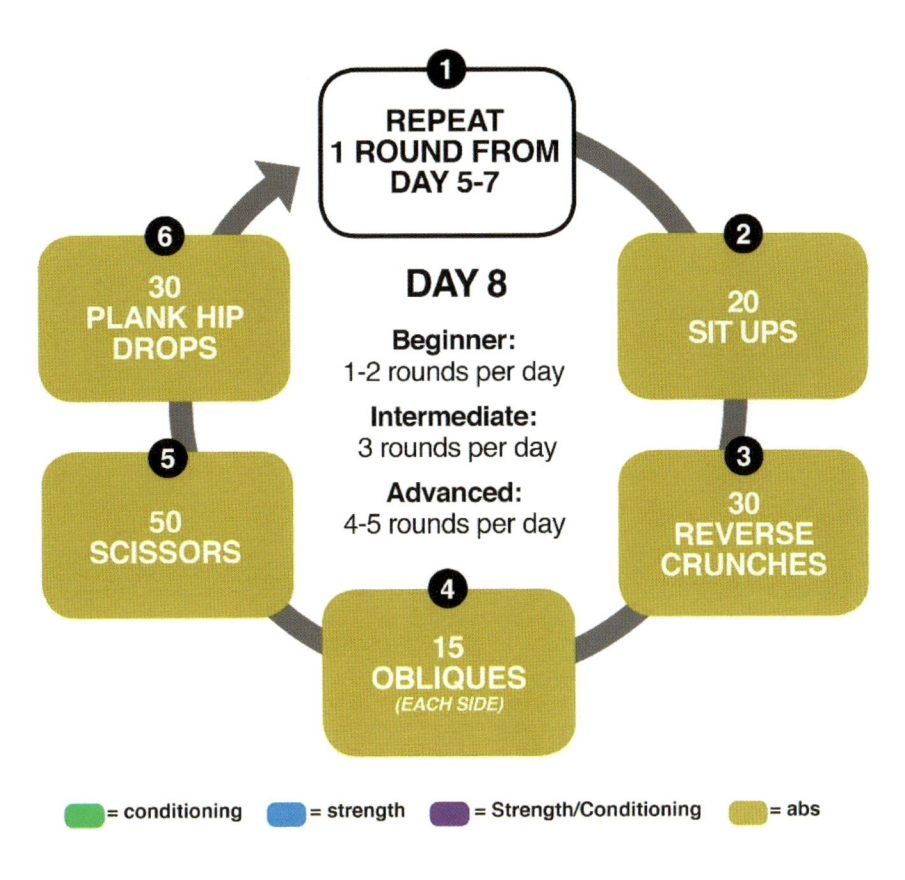

DAY 8

Beginner: 1-2 rounds per day

Intermediate: 3 rounds per day

Advanced: 4-5 rounds per day

1. REPEAT 1 ROUND FROM DAY 5-7
2. 20 SIT UPS
3. 30 REVERSE CRUNCHES
4. 15 OBLIQUES (EACH SIDE)
5. 50 SCISSORS
6. 30 PLANK HIP DROPS

- = conditioning
- = strength
- = Strength/Conditioning
- = abs

Warm up prior to workout http://bit.ly/10YPaIU

Bonus Video-Tutorial Day 8 http://bit.ly/Zvgtx2

31 DAYS OF FAT BURNING WORKOUTS

DAY 9

MOTIVATION

Your perfect time will never come, don't wait, work out today.

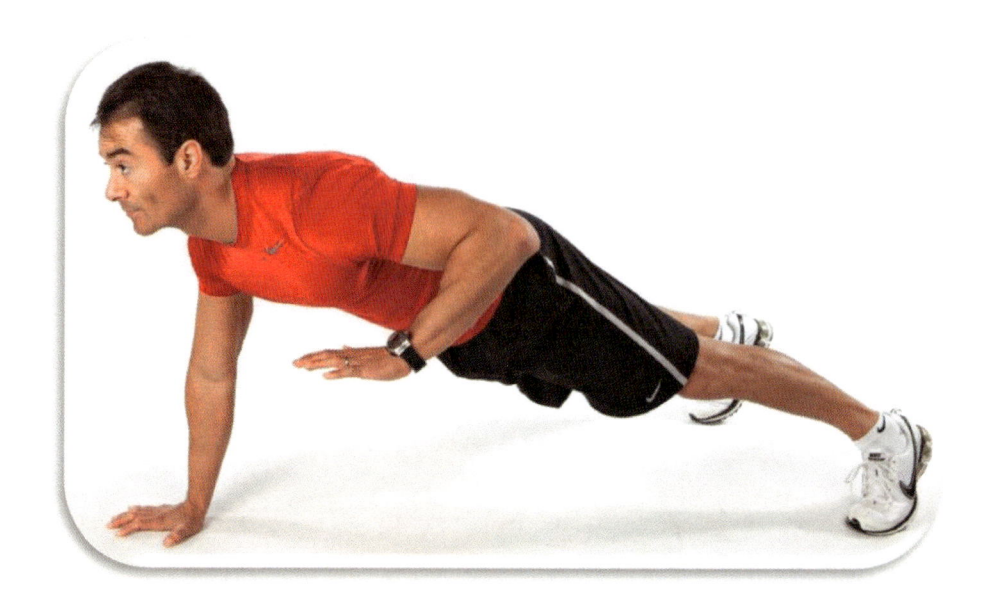

HEALTHY EATING TIP

Ask for salad dressings to be served "on the side", so you can add only as much as you need.

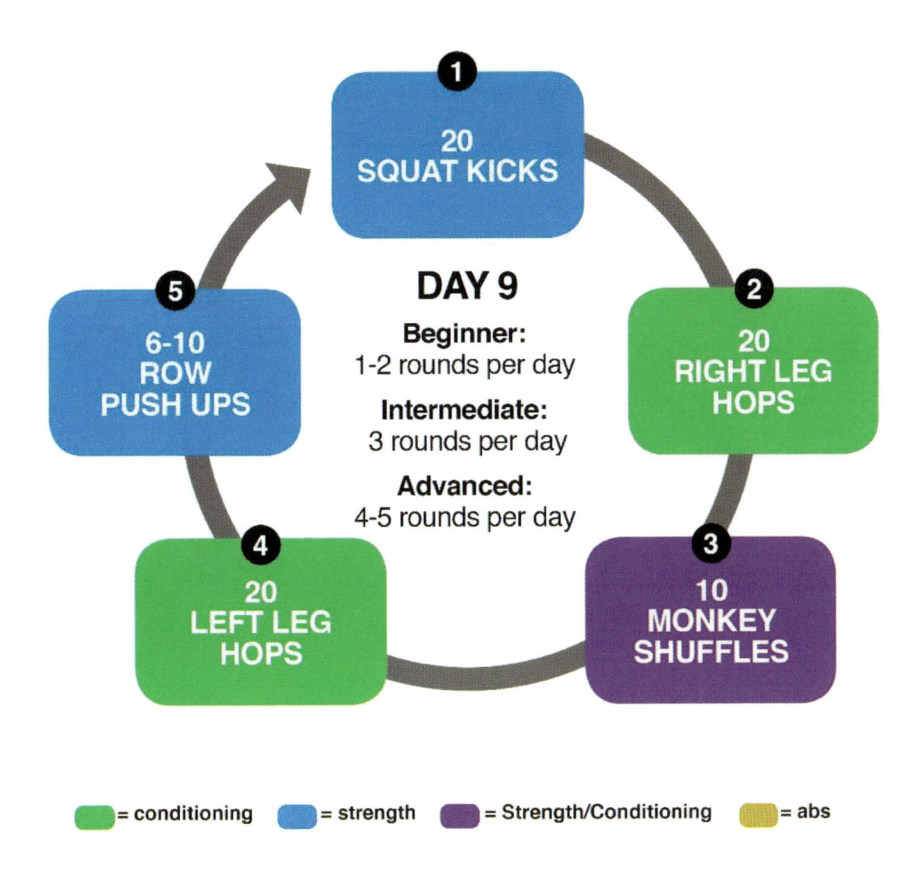

DAY 9

Beginner: 1-2 rounds per day

Intermediate: 3 rounds per day

Advanced: 4-5 rounds per day

1. 20 SQUAT KICKS
2. 20 RIGHT LEG HOPS
3. 10 MONKEY SHUFFLES
4. 20 LEFT LEG HOPS
5. 6-10 ROW PUSH UPS

- = conditioning
- = strength
- = Strength/Conditioning
- = abs

Warm up prior to workout http://bit.ly/10YPaIU

Bonus Video-Tutorial Day 9 http://bit.ly/Y8ioXo

DAY 10

MOTIVATION

The results are closer than you think.

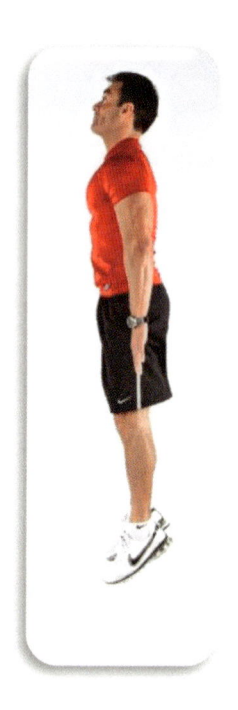

HEALTHY EATING TIP

Replace mayonnaise and sour cream with non-fat Greek yogurt to minimize calories.

31 DAYS OF FAT BURNING WORKOUTS

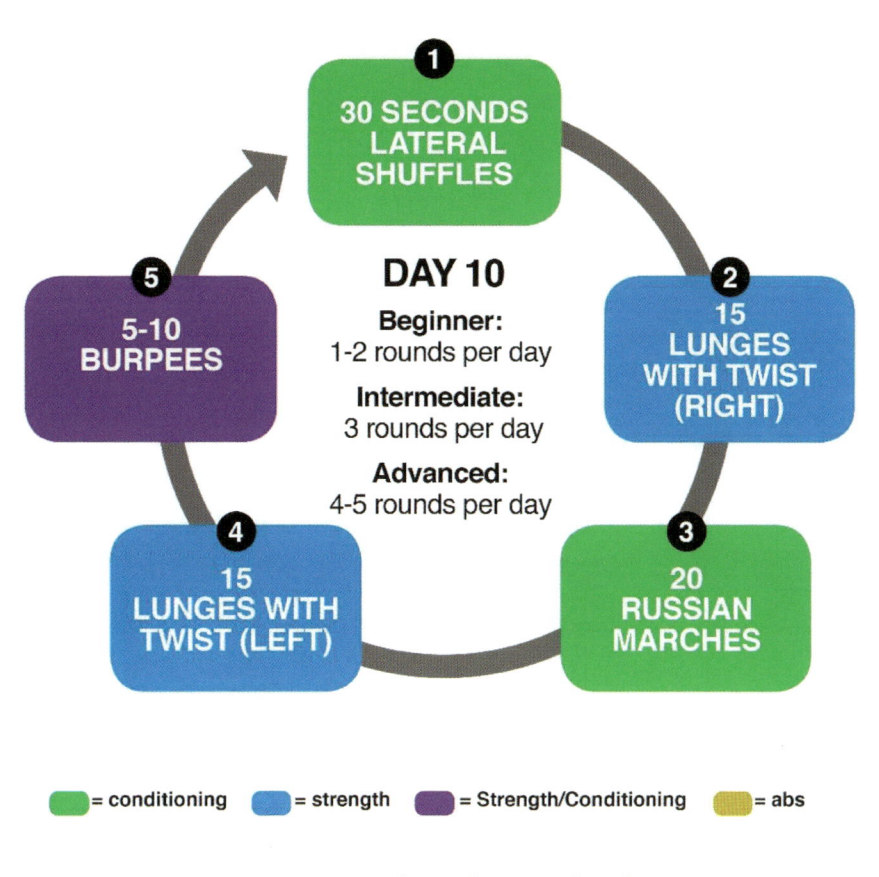

DAY 10

1. 30 SECONDS LATERAL SHUFFLES

2. 15 LUNGES WITH TWIST (RIGHT)

3. 20 RUSSIAN MARCHES

4. 15 LUNGES WITH TWIST (LEFT)

5. 5-10 BURPEES

Beginner: 1-2 rounds per day
Intermediate: 3 rounds per day
Advanced: 4-5 rounds per day

- = conditioning
- = strength
- = Strength/Conditioning
- = abs

Warm up prior to workout http://bit.ly/10YPaIU

Bonus Video-Tutorial Day 10 http://bit.ly/11wsdgH

31 DAYS OF FAT BURNING WORKOUTS

DAY 11

MOTIVATION

Your dream body cannot be built in one day, be patient.

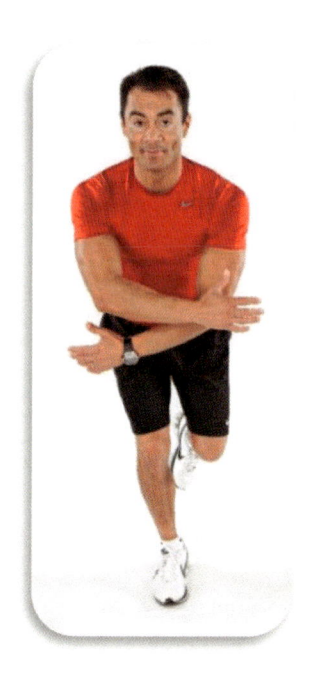

HEALTHY EATING TIP

Keep a bowl of whole fruit on the table, counter, or in the refrigerator to remind you to eat a healthy snack.

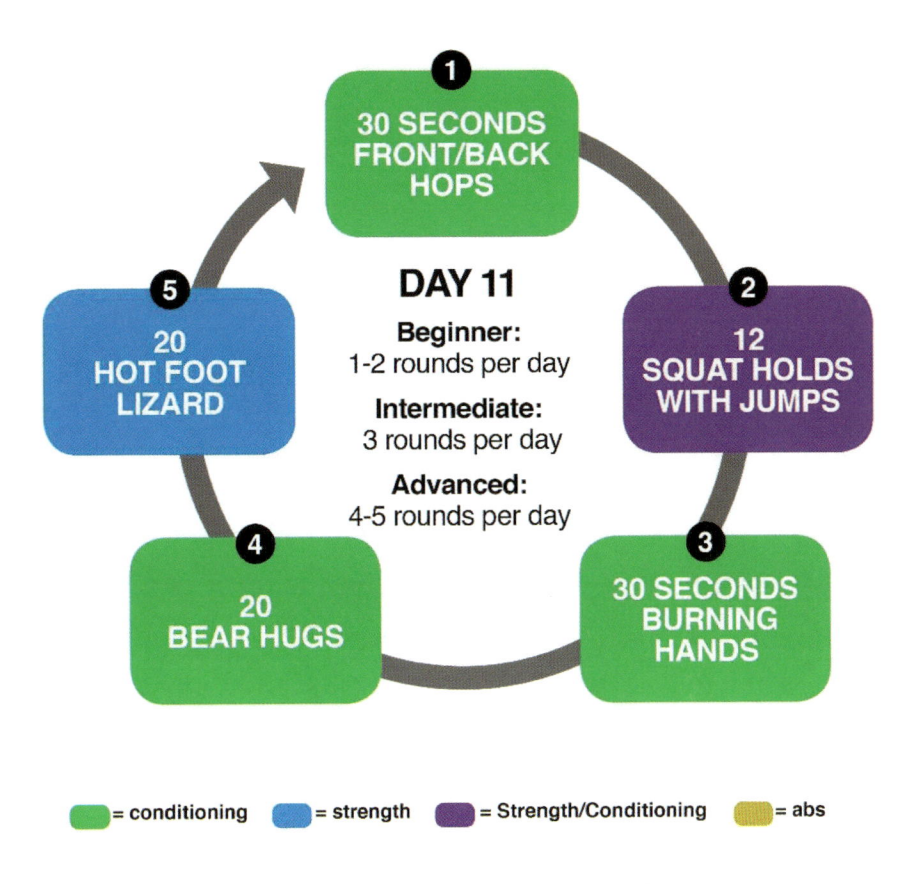

DAY 11

1 30 SECONDS FRONT/BACK HOPS

2 12 SQUAT HOLDS WITH JUMPS

3 30 SECONDS BURNING HANDS

4 20 BEAR HUGS

5 20 HOT FOOT LIZARD

Beginner: 1-2 rounds per day

Intermediate: 3 rounds per day

Advanced: 4-5 rounds per day

- = conditioning
- = strength
- = Strength/Conditioning
- = abs

Warm up prior to workout http://bit.ly/10YPaIU

Bonus Video-Tutorial Day 11 http://bit.ly/YgvqUZ

DAY 12

MOTIVATION

Bored muscles don't work, confuse your muscles and they will.

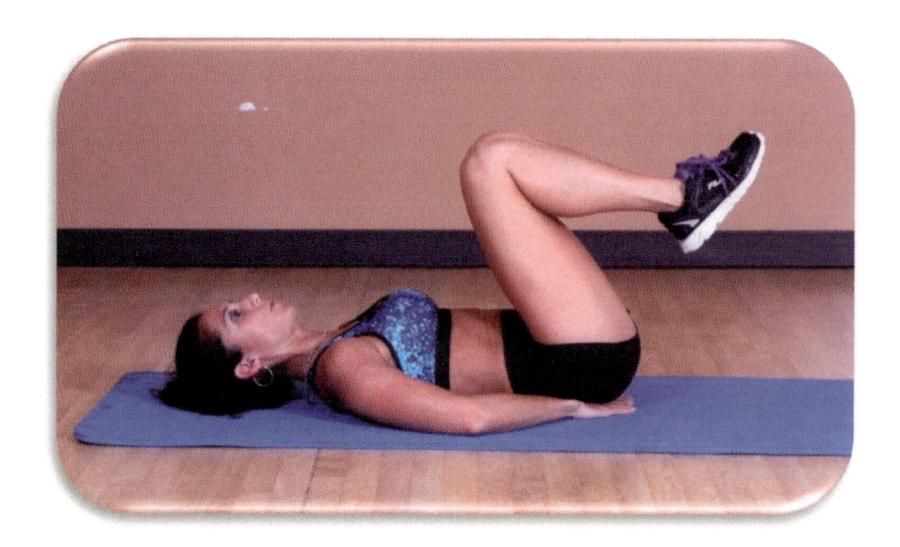

HEALTHY EATING TIP

Switch high calorie breakfast choices like bagels with cream cheese and juice for lower calorie items like sugar-free oatmeal and cooked egg whites.

31 DAYS OF FAT BURNING WORKOUTS

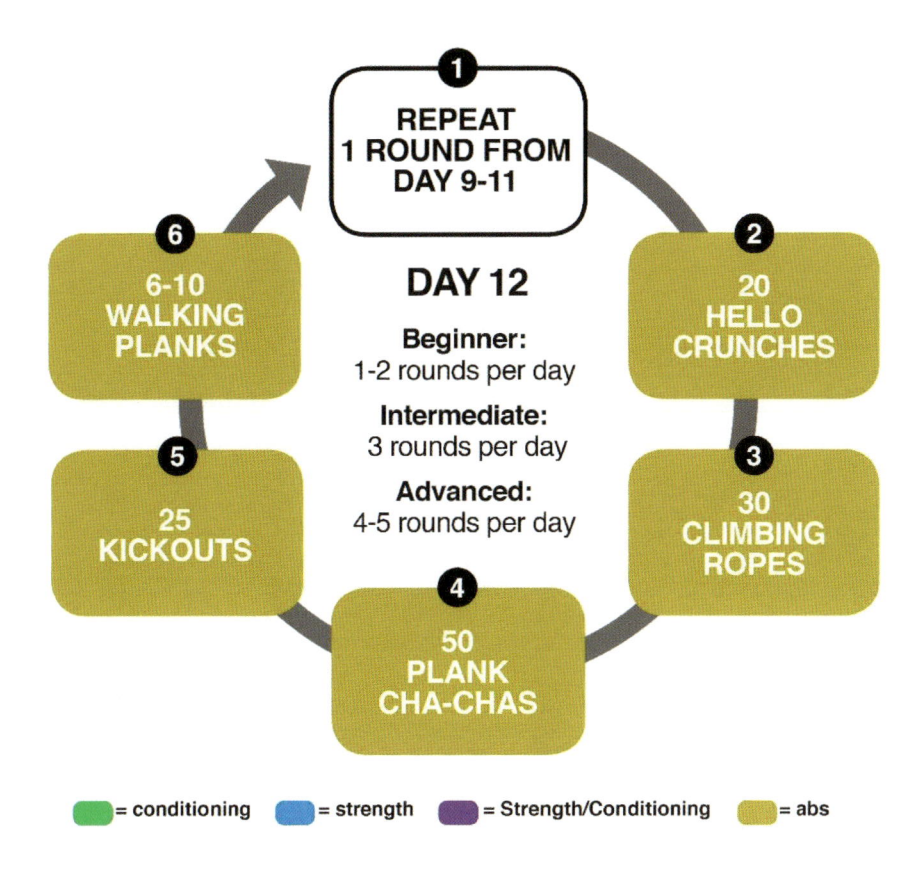

DAY 12

Beginner: 1-2 rounds per day

Intermediate: 3 rounds per day

Advanced: 4-5 rounds per day

1. REPEAT 1 ROUND FROM DAY 9-11
2. 20 HELLO CRUNCHES
3. 30 CLIMBING ROPES
4. 50 PLANK CHA-CHAS
5. 25 KICKOUTS
6. 6-10 WALKING PLANKS

= conditioning   = strength   = Strength/Conditioning   = abs

Warm up prior to workout http://bit.ly/10YPaIU

Bonus Video-Tutorial Day 12 http://bit.ly/16t4FiC

31 DAYS OF FAT BURNING WORKOUTS

DAY 13

MOTIVATION

Stay hungry for more, never less.

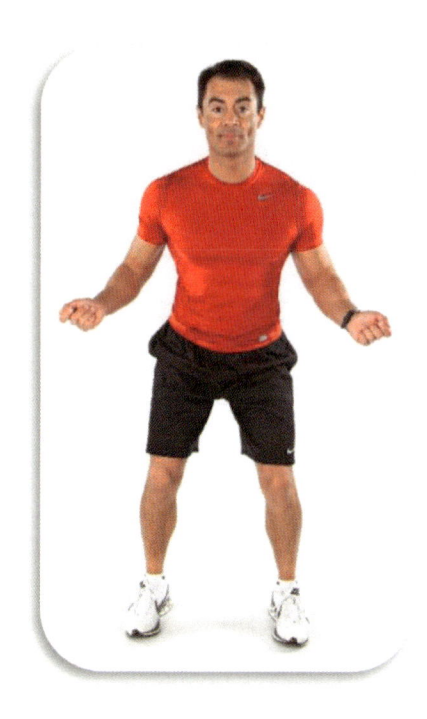

HEALTHY EATING TIP

Create a new habit by replacing beverages high in sugar with water.

31 DAYS OF FAT BURNING WORKOUTS

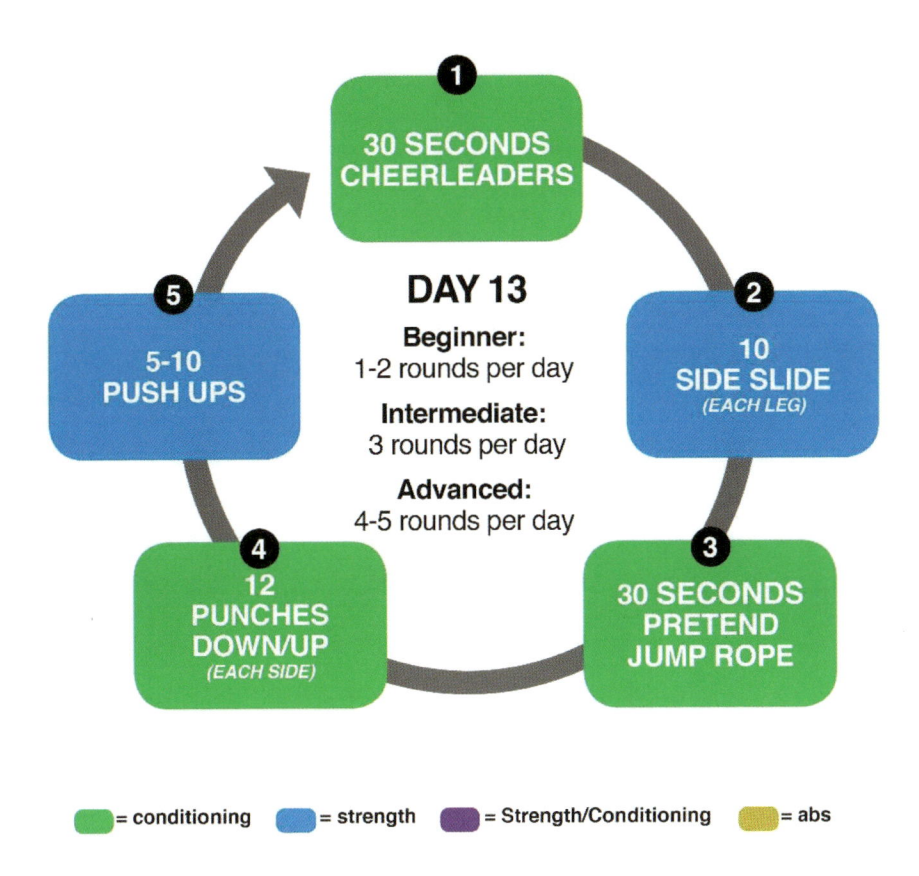

DAY 13

1. 30 SECONDS CHEERLEADERS

2. 10 SIDE SLIDE (EACH LEG)

3. 30 SECONDS PRETEND JUMP ROPE

4. 12 PUNCHES DOWN/UP (EACH SIDE)

5. 5-10 PUSH UPS

Beginner: 1-2 rounds per day
Intermediate: 3 rounds per day
Advanced: 4-5 rounds per day

■ = conditioning ■ = strength ■ = Strength/Conditioning ■ = abs

Warm up prior to workout http://bit.ly/10YPaIU

Bonus Video-Tutorial Day 13 http://bit.ly/15bJ4Mu

- 45 -

31 DAYS OF FAT BURNING WORKOUTS

DAY 14

MOTIVATION

Live, learn, love, and work out. Repeat!

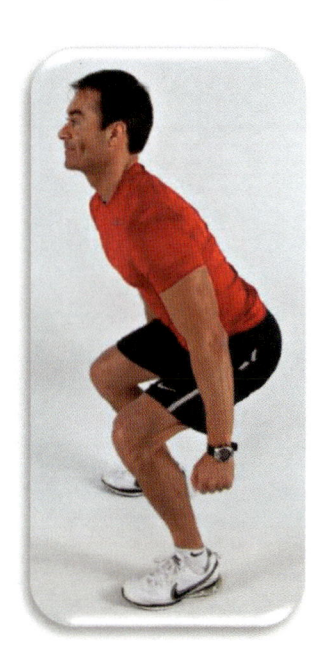

HEALTHY EATING TIP

Divide large restaurant portions in half when dining out. By taking half of your meal home you will consume fewer calories and have an extra meal.

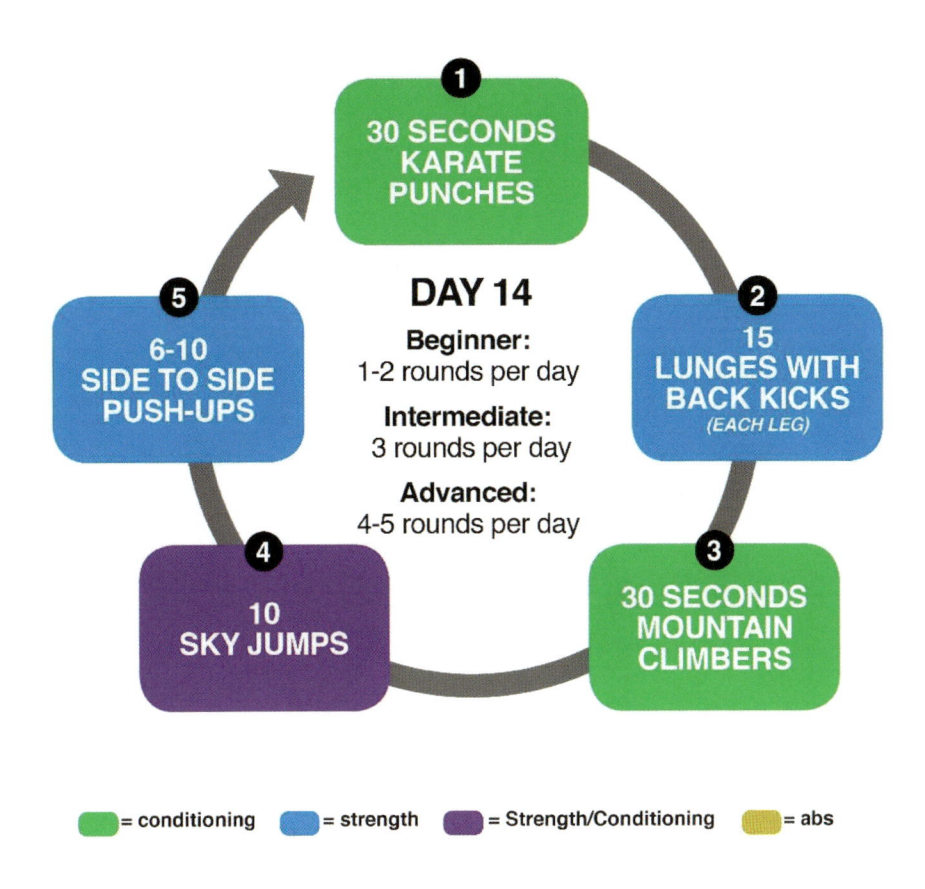

DAY 14

Beginner: 1-2 rounds per day

Intermediate: 3 rounds per day

Advanced: 4-5 rounds per day

1. 30 SECONDS KARATE PUNCHES
2. 15 LUNGES WITH BACK KICKS (EACH LEG)
3. 30 SECONDS MOUNTAIN CLIMBERS
4. 10 SKY JUMPS
5. 6-10 SIDE TO SIDE PUSH-UPS

- = conditioning
- = strength
- = Strength/Conditioning
- = abs

Warm up prior to workout http://bit.ly/10YPaIU

Bonus Video-Tutorial Day 14 http://bit.ly/12oBFcN

DAY 15

MOTIVATION

Everything starts in your mind, PUSH and your body will follow.

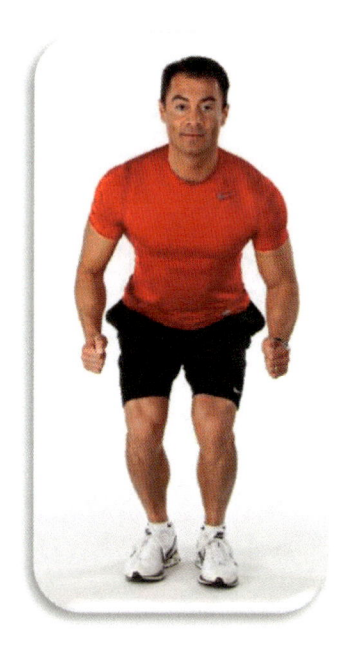

HEALTHY EATING TIP

Eat slowly; it takes about 20 minutes for the stomach to tell the brain that it is full.

31 DAYS OF FAT BURNING WORKOUTS

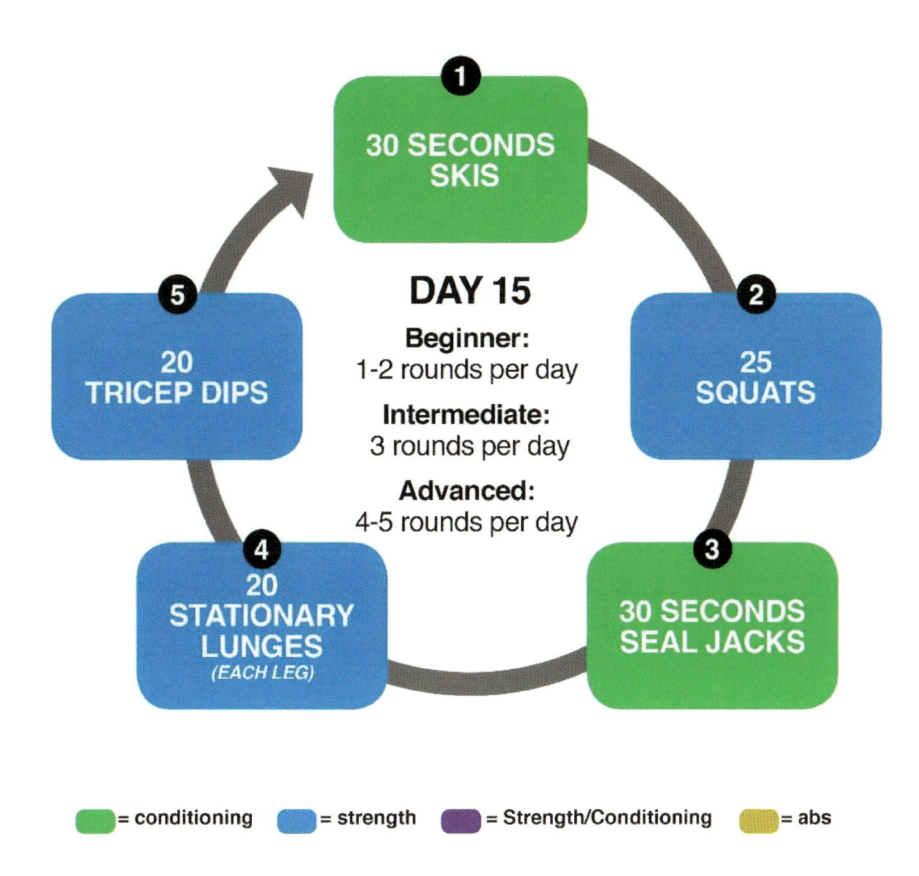

DAY 15

1. 30 SECONDS SKIS
2. 25 SQUATS
3. 30 SECONDS SEAL JACKS
4. 20 STATIONARY LUNGES (EACH LEG)
5. 20 TRICEP DIPS

Beginner: 1-2 rounds per day

Intermediate: 3 rounds per day

Advanced: 4-5 rounds per day

- = conditioning
- = strength
- = Strength/Conditioning
- = abs

Warm up prior to workout http://bit.ly/10YPaIU

Bonus Video-Tutorial Day 15 http://bit.ly/10iBs5X

31 DAYS OF FAT BURNING WORKOUTS

DAY 16

MOTIVATION

Think, act and work out like a champ, because you are.

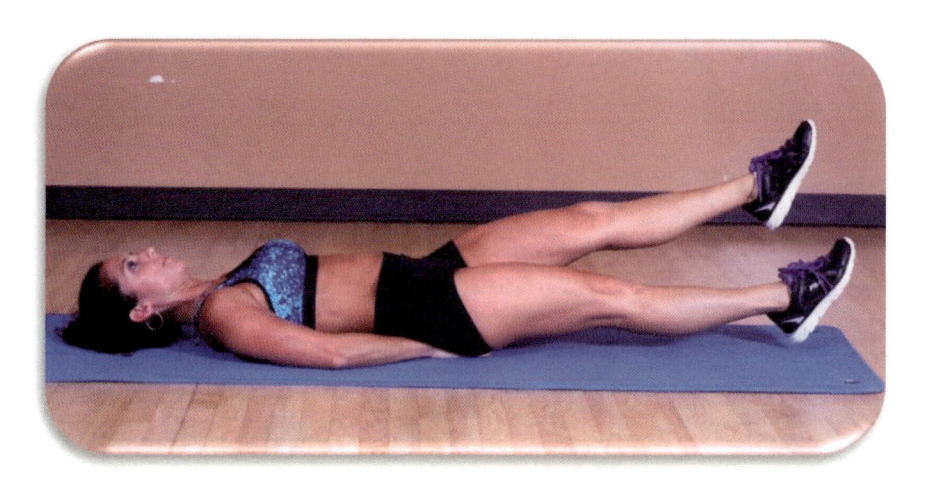

HEALTHY EATING TIP

Take control of your calorie intake by not eating in front of the TV or while surfing on the internet.

DAY 16

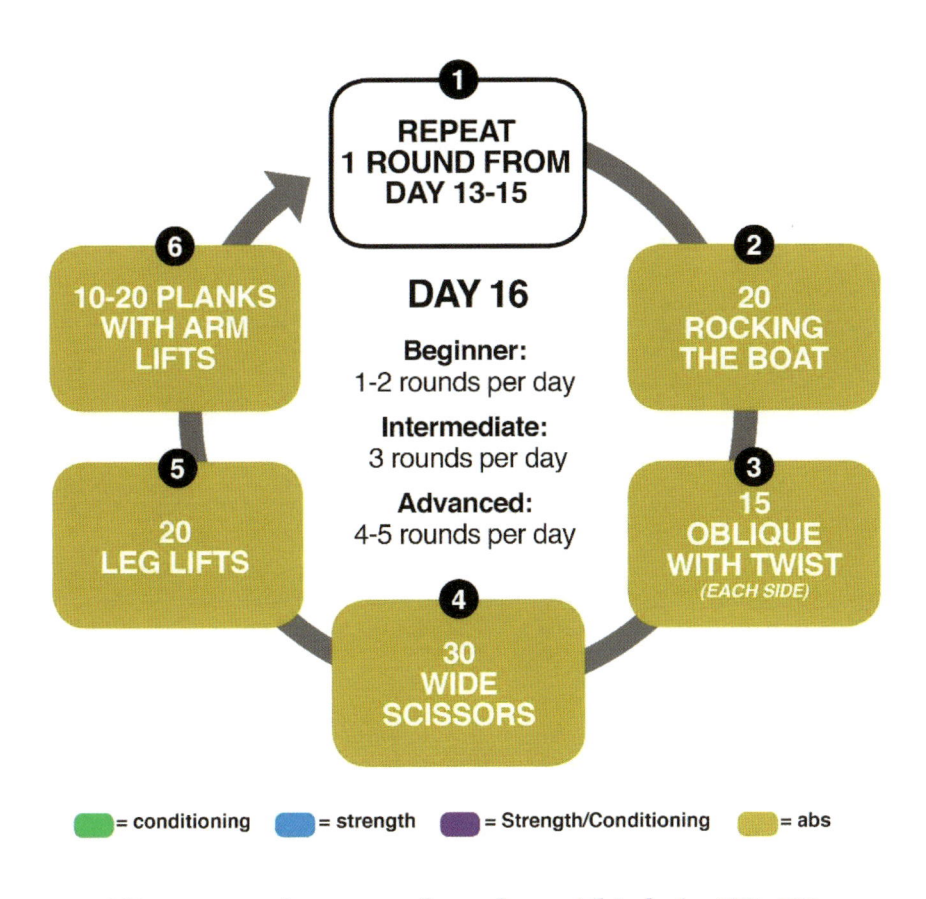

Beginner: 1-2 rounds per day

Intermediate: 3 rounds per day

Advanced: 4-5 rounds per day

1. REPEAT 1 ROUND FROM DAY 13-15
2. 20 ROCKING THE BOAT
3. 15 OBLIQUE WITH TWIST *(EACH SIDE)*
4. 30 WIDE SCISSORS
5. 20 LEG LIFTS
6. 10-20 PLANKS WITH ARM LIFTS

🟢 = conditioning 🔵 = strength 🟣 = Strength/Conditioning 🟡 = abs

Warm up prior to workout http://bit.ly/10YPaIU

Bonus Video-Tutorial Day 16 http://bit.ly/19cFqOH

31 DAYS OF FAT BURNING WORKOUTS

DAY 17

MOTIVATION

Positive thinking, positive results.

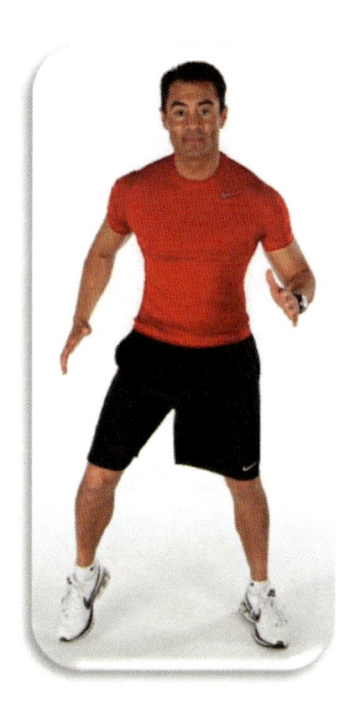

HEALTHY EATING TIP

Replace fried foods with baked, poached, roasted or grilled foods.

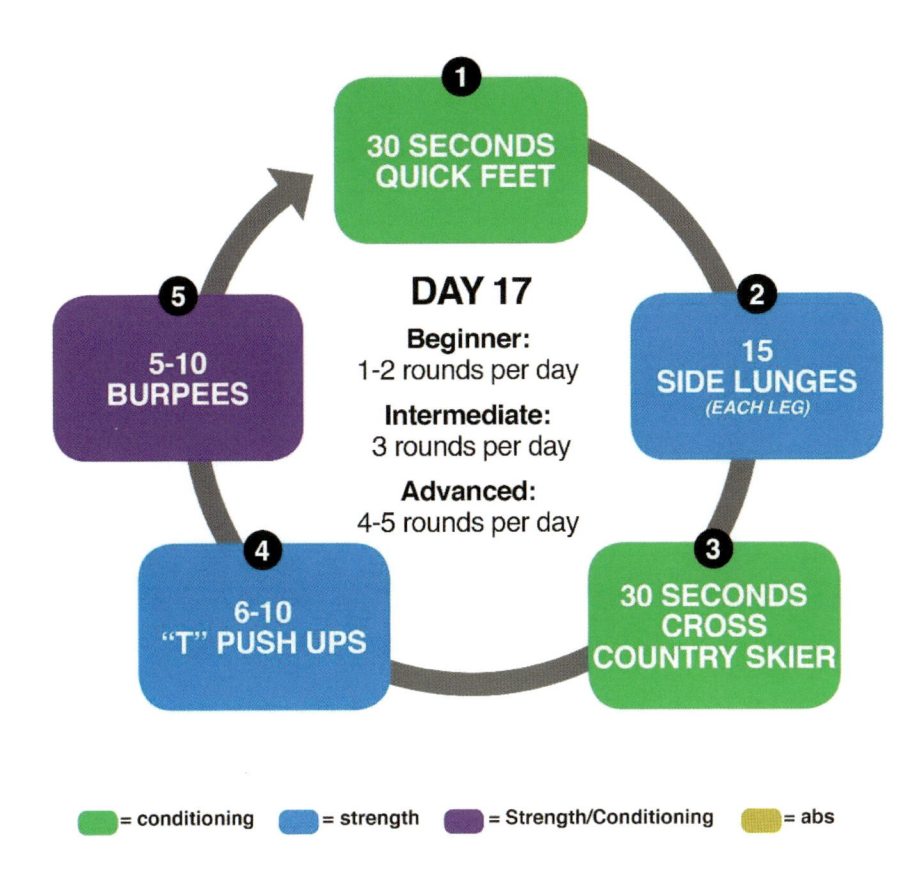

DAY 17

Beginner: 1-2 rounds per day
Intermediate: 3 rounds per day
Advanced: 4-5 rounds per day

1. 30 SECONDS QUICK FEET
2. 15 SIDE LUNGES (EACH LEG)
3. 30 SECONDS CROSS COUNTRY SKIER
4. 6-10 "T" PUSH UPS
5. 5-10 BURPEES

■ = conditioning   ■ = strength   ■ = Strength/Conditioning   ■ = abs

Warm up prior to workout http://bit.ly/10YPaIU

Bonus Video-Tutorial Day 17 http://bit.ly/17eQvSQ

DAY 18

MOTIVATION

Be fearless to any new challenge, your body will adapt.

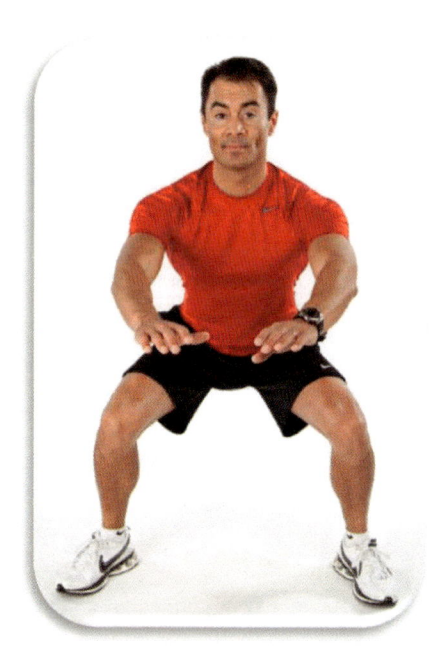

HEALTHY EATING TIP

Do not skip breakfast or lunch; you still have a long day ahead and your body needs nutrients to keep your metabolism going.

31 DAYS OF FAT BURNING WORKOUTS

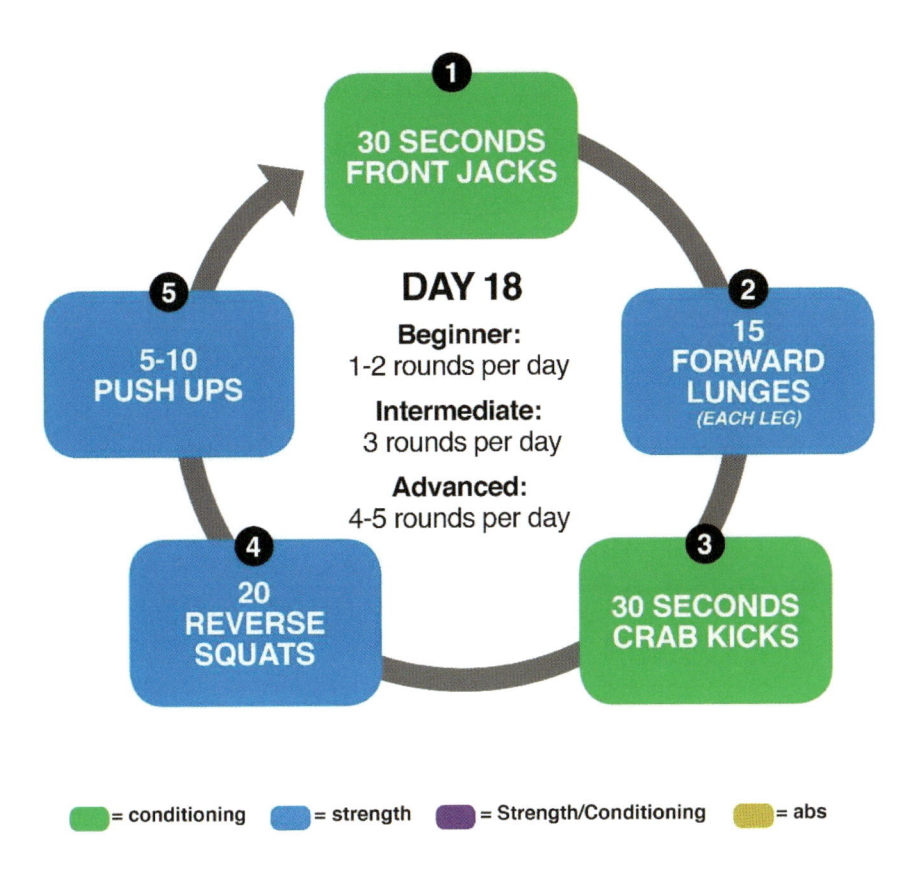

DAY 18

1. 30 SECONDS FRONT JACKS
2. 15 FORWARD LUNGES (EACH LEG)
3. 30 SECONDS CRAB KICKS
4. 20 REVERSE SQUATS
5. 5-10 PUSH UPS

Beginner: 1-2 rounds per day
Intermediate: 3 rounds per day
Advanced: 4-5 rounds per day

■ = conditioning   ■ = strength   ■ = Strength/Conditioning   ■ = abs

Warm up prior to workout http://bit.ly/1oYPaIU

Bonus Video-Tutorial Day 18 http://bit.ly/19cFIVR

- 55 -

31 DAYS OF FAT BURNING WORKOUTS

DAY 19

MOTIVATION

No obstacles will hold you back if you make a plan to overcome them.

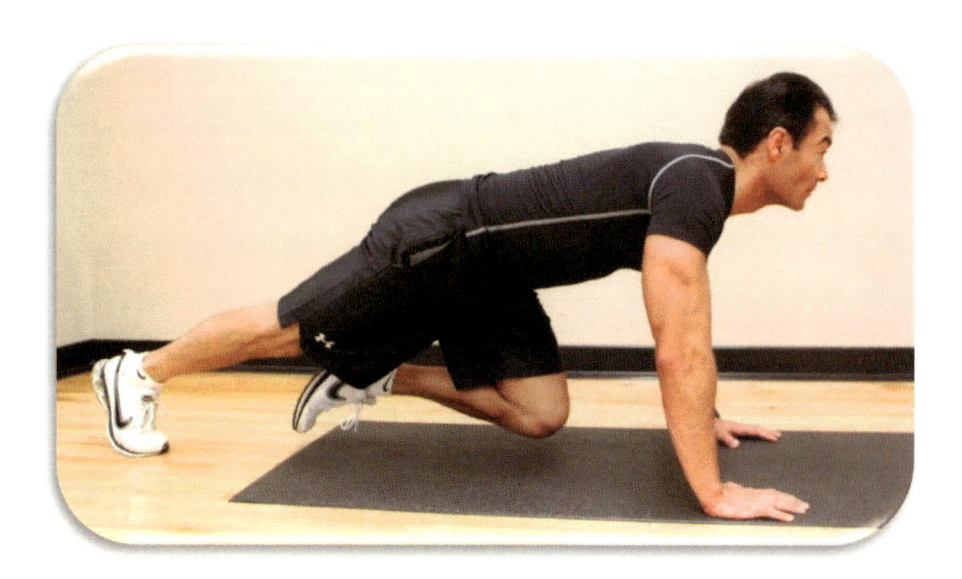

HEALTHY EATING TIP

Avoid the temptation of having treats in the house; enjoy them in small portions away from home.

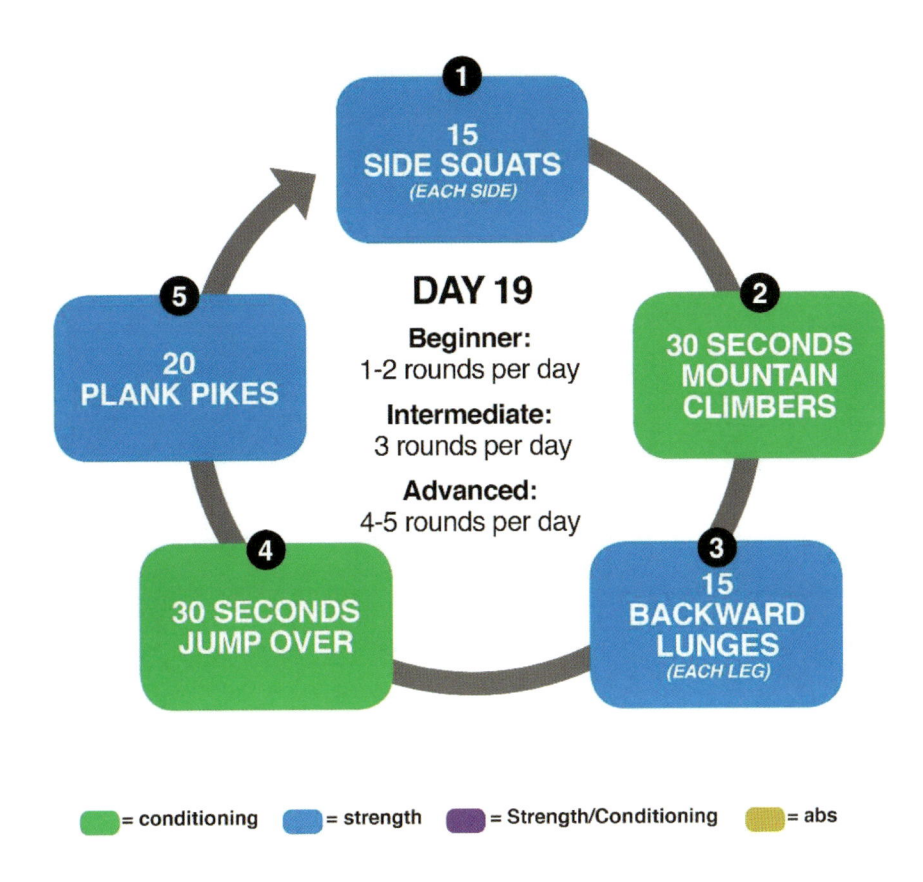

DAY 19

Beginner: 1-2 rounds per day

Intermediate: 3 rounds per day

Advanced: 4-5 rounds per day

1. 15 SIDE SQUATS (EACH SIDE)
2. 30 SECONDS MOUNTAIN CLIMBERS
3. 15 BACKWARD LUNGES (EACH LEG)
4. 30 SECONDS JUMP OVER
5. 20 PLANK PIKES

= conditioning   = strength   = Strength/Conditioning   = abs

Warm up prior to workout http://bit.ly/10YPaIU

Bonus Video-Tutorial Day 19 http://bit.ly/10DLa4H

31 DAYS OF FAT BURNING WORKOUTS

DAY 20

MOTIVATION

Every workout builds energy and energy will build you.

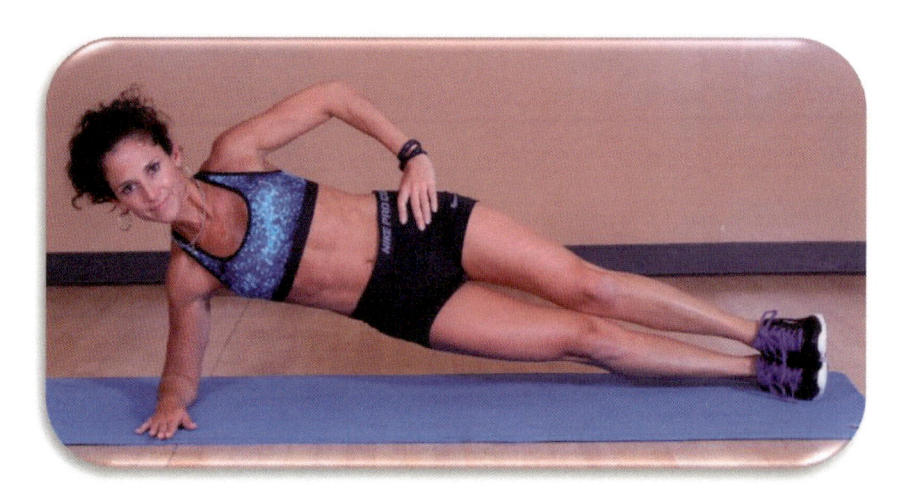

HEALTHY EATING TIP

Eating foods high in fiber like beans, lentils and edamame, will keep you full longer and will help to burn more calories.

DAY 20

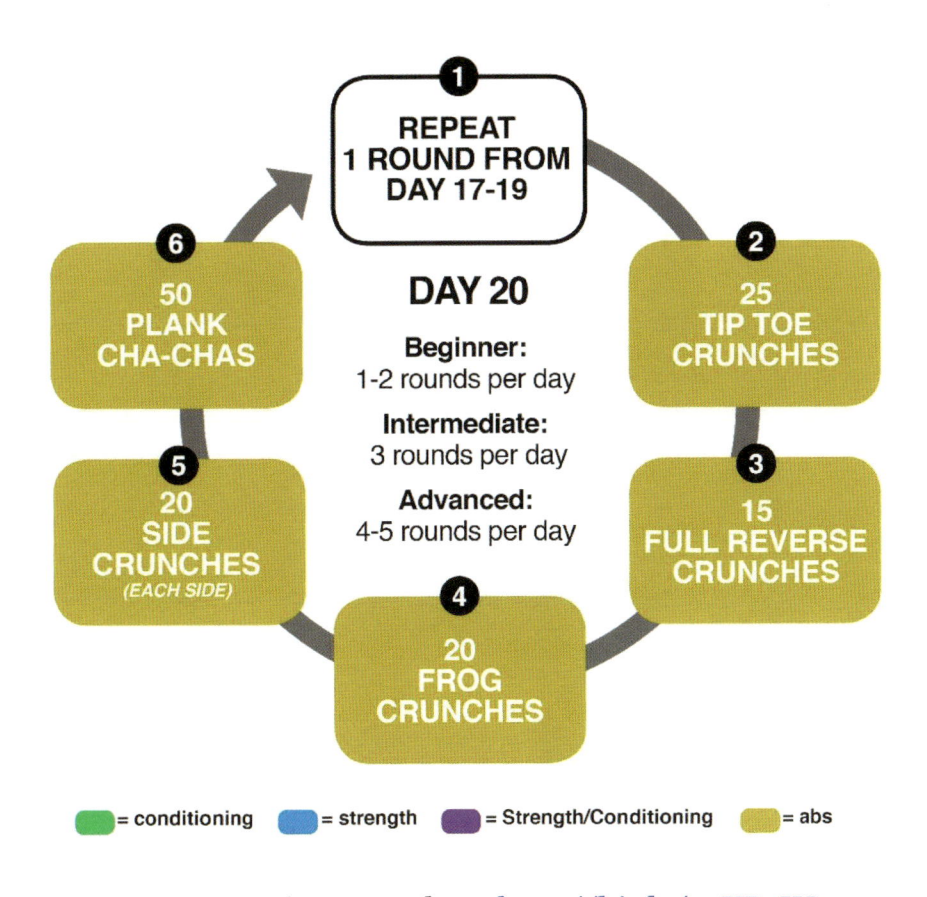

Beginner: 1-2 rounds per day

Intermediate: 3 rounds per day

Advanced: 4-5 rounds per day

1. REPEAT 1 ROUND FROM DAY 17-19
2. 25 TIP TOE CRUNCHES
3. 15 FULL REVERSE CRUNCHES
4. 20 FROG CRUNCHES
5. 20 SIDE CRUNCHES (EACH SIDE)
6. 50 PLANK CHA-CHAS

- 🟢 = conditioning
- 🔵 = strength
- 🟣 = Strength/Conditioning
- 🟡 = abs

Warm up prior to workout http://bit.ly/10YPaIU

Bonus Video-Tutorial Day 20 http://bit.ly/13O4z1N

31 DAYS OF FAT BURNING WORKOUTS

DAY 21

MOTIVATION

Don't think about it, just get your workout done.

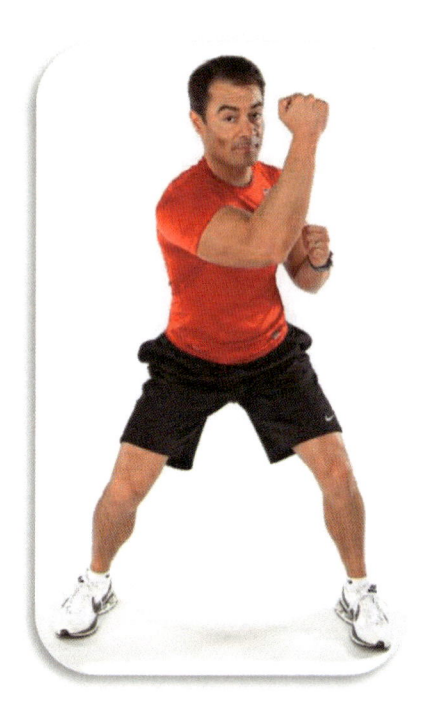

HEALTHY EATING TIP

Consider low-fat alternatives to whole milk, like reduced fat milk or soy milk.

DAY 21

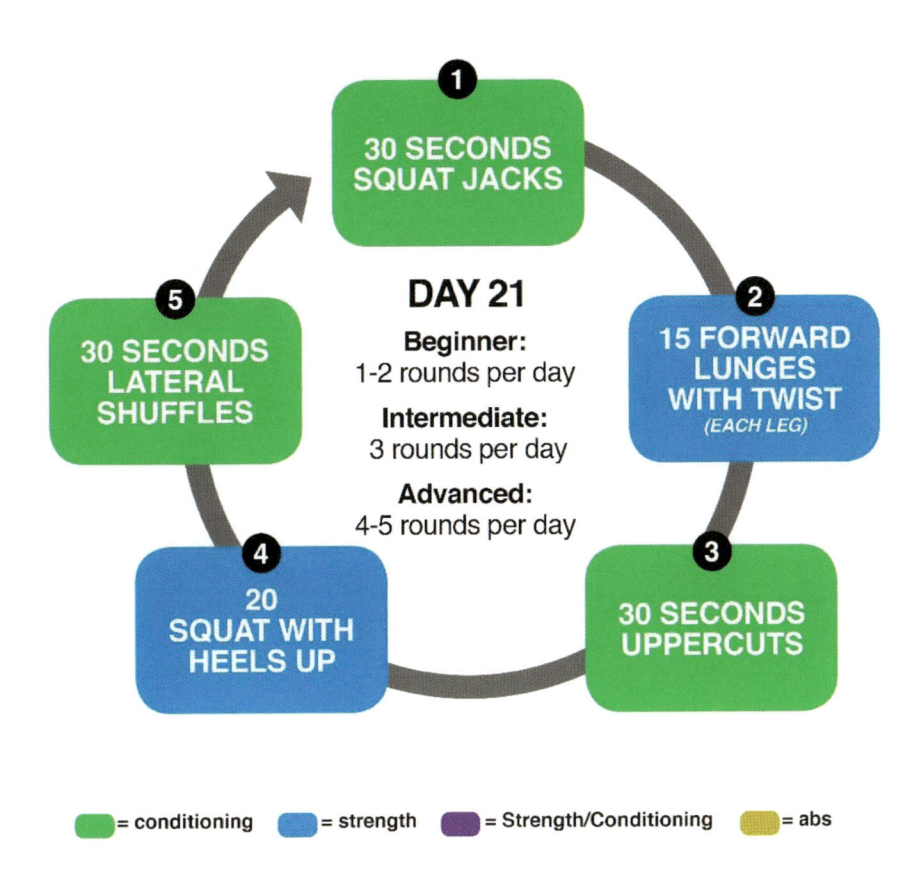

Beginner: 1-2 rounds per day

Intermediate: 3 rounds per day

Advanced: 4-5 rounds per day

1. 30 SECONDS SQUAT JACKS
2. 15 FORWARD LUNGES WITH TWIST (EACH LEG)
3. 30 SECONDS UPPERCUTS
4. 20 SQUAT WITH HEELS UP
5. 30 SECONDS LATERAL SHUFFLES

= conditioning   = strength   = Strength/Conditioning   = abs

Warm up prior to workout http://bit.ly/10YPaIU

Bonus Video-Tutorial Day 21 http://bit.ly/10zpi6f

31 DAYS OF FAT BURNING WORKOUTS

DAY 22

MOTIVATION

Feeling happy, work out; feeling down, work out; in doubt, keep working out!

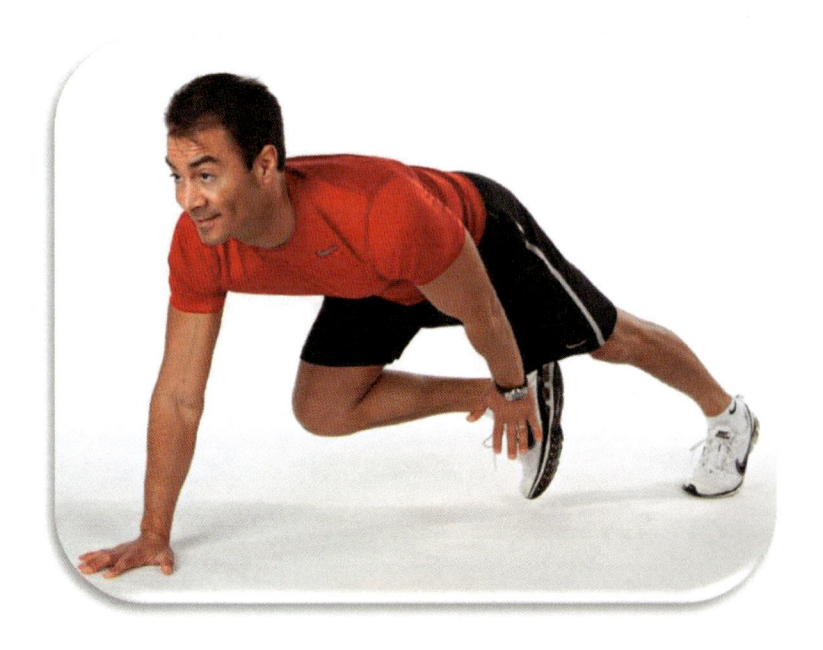

HEALTHY EATING TIP

Eat a small healthy meal before exercise (carbs preferred) to fuel your body and increase your energy level.

31 DAYS OF FAT BURNING WORKOUTS

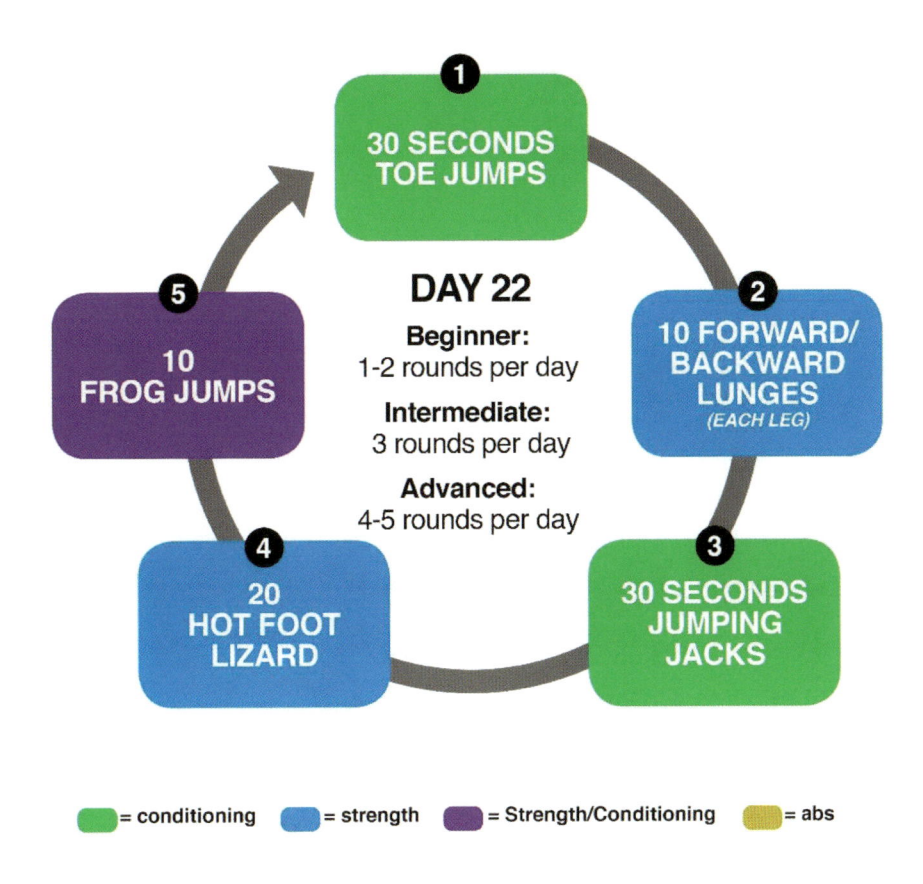

DAY 22

1. 30 SECONDS TOE JUMPS
2. 10 FORWARD/BACKWARD LUNGES (EACH LEG)
3. 30 SECONDS JUMPING JACKS
4. 20 HOT FOOT LIZARD
5. 10 FROG JUMPS

Beginner: 1-2 rounds per day
Intermediate: 3 rounds per day
Advanced: 4-5 rounds per day

- = conditioning
- = strength
- = Strength/Conditioning
- = abs

Warm up prior to workout http://bit.ly/10YPaIU

Bonus Video-Tutorial Day 22 http://bit.ly/11pd7oE

31 DAYS OF FAT BURNING WORKOUTS

DAY 23

MOTIVATION

"I cannot" is useless, erase it, and start saying "YES I CAN".

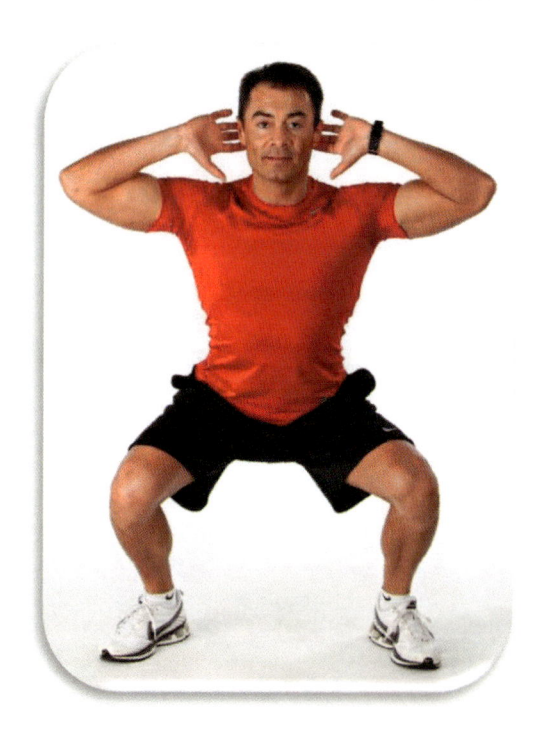

HEALTHY EATING TIP

When dining out, choose menu items that are grilled, baked, steamed, or roasted.

DAY 23

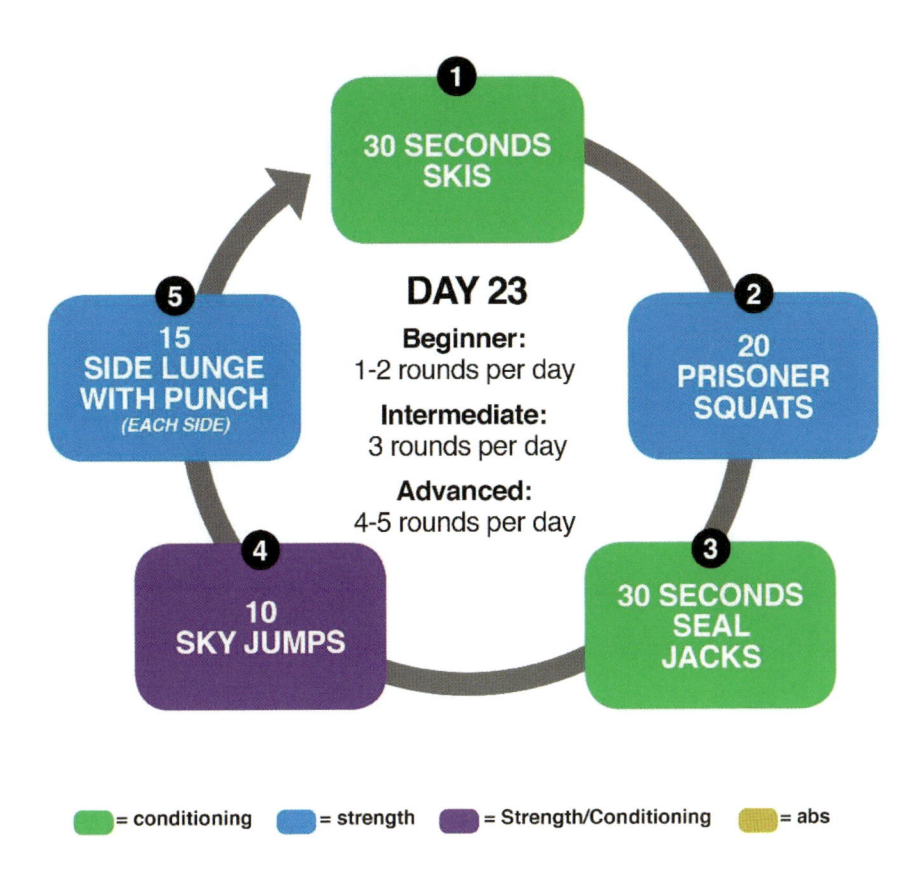

Beginner: 1-2 rounds per day

Intermediate: 3 rounds per day

Advanced: 4-5 rounds per day

1. 30 SECONDS SKIS
2. 20 PRISONER SQUATS
3. 30 SECONDS SEAL JACKS
4. 10 SKY JUMPS
5. 15 SIDE LUNGE WITH PUNCH (EACH SIDE)

■ = conditioning   ■ = strength   ■ = Strength/Conditioning   ■ = abs

Warm up prior to workout http://bit.ly/10YPaIU

Bonus Video-Tutorial Day 23 http://bit.ly/Z8Olzh

31 DAYS OF FAT BURNING WORKOUTS

DAY 24

MOTIVATION

Think about reaching your goal, not being perfect.

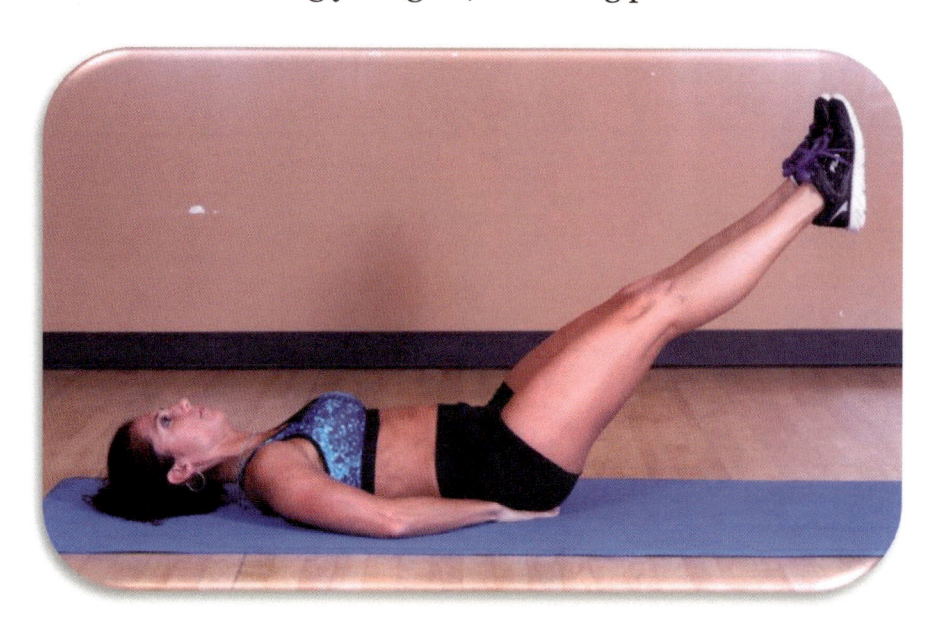

HEALTHY EATING TIP

Pack a healthy lunch from home when possible; you will eat a healthier meal and spend less money on take-out food.

31 DAYS OF FAT BURNING WORKOUTS

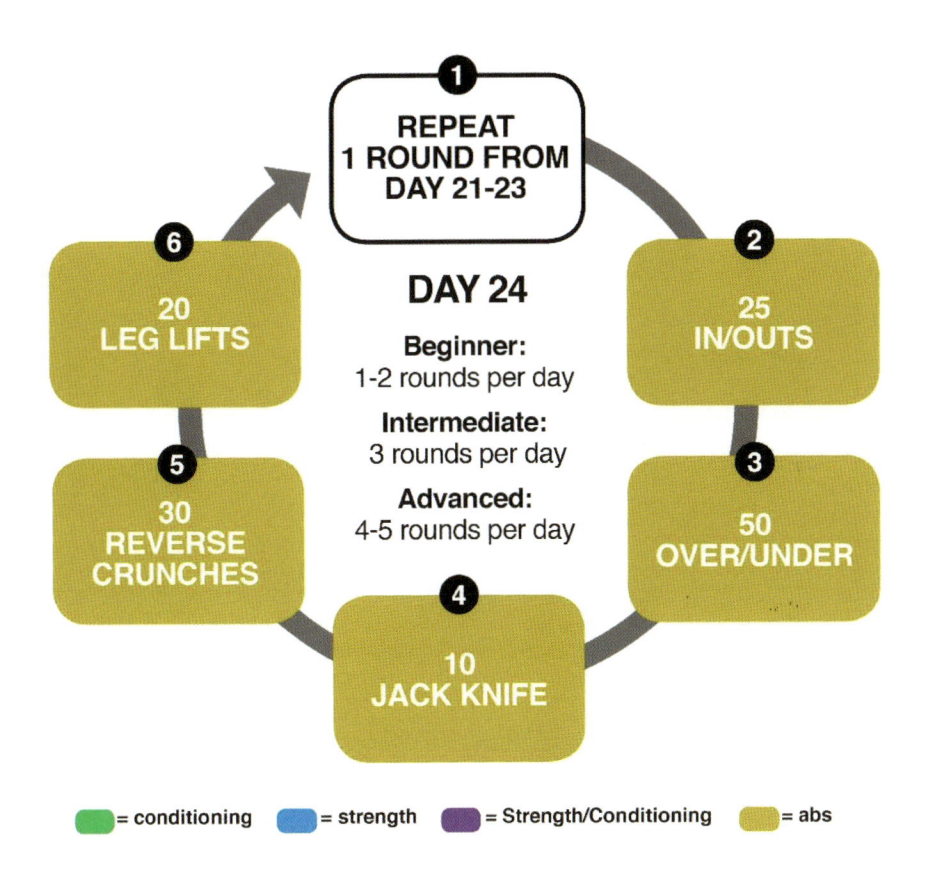

1. REPEAT 1 ROUND FROM DAY 21-23

2. 25 IN/OUTS

3. 50 OVER/UNDER

4. 10 JACK KNIFE

5. 30 REVERSE CRUNCHES

6. 20 LEG LIFTS

DAY 24

Beginner: 1-2 rounds per day

Intermediate: 3 rounds per day

Advanced: 4-5 rounds per day

= conditioning   = strength   = Strength/Conditioning   = abs

Warm up prior to workout http://bit.ly/10YPaIU

Bonus Video-Tutorial Day 24 http://bit.ly/11pdnwF

31 DAYS OF FAT BURNING WORKOUTS

DAY 25

MOTIVATION

Your mind and body are very powerful, marry them.

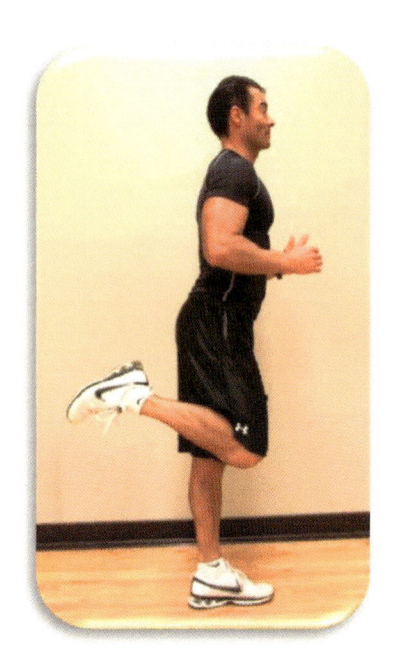

HEALTHY EATING TIP

Minimize your consumption of sugar and your cravings will begin to disappear; sugar is addictive and it is hidden everywhere.

31 DAYS OF FAT BURNING WORKOUTS

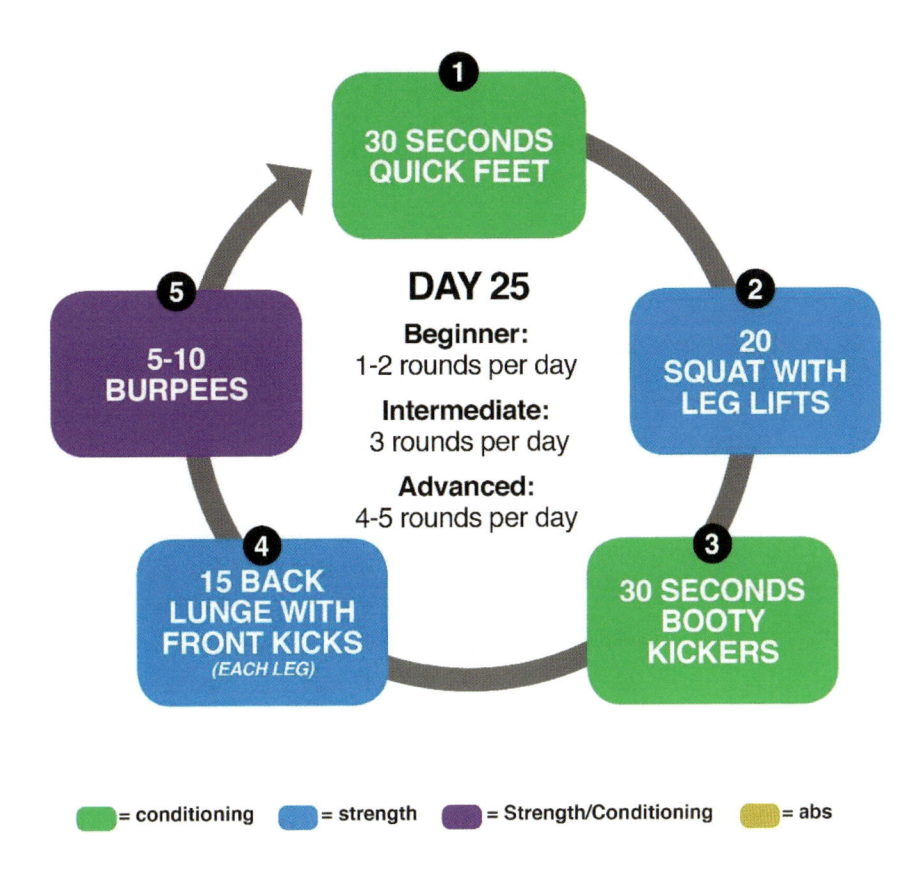

DAY 25

Beginner: 1-2 rounds per day
Intermediate: 3 rounds per day
Advanced: 4-5 rounds per day

1. 30 SECONDS QUICK FEET
2. 20 SQUAT WITH LEG LIFTS
3. 30 SECONDS BOOTY KICKERS
4. 15 BACK LUNGE WITH FRONT KICKS (EACH LEG)
5. 5-10 BURPEES

- = conditioning
- = strength
- = Strength/Conditioning
- = abs

Warm up prior to workout http://bit.ly/10YPaIU

Bonus Video-Tutorial Day 25 http://bit.ly/112e89R

31 DAYS OF FAT BURNING WORKOUTS

DAY 26

MOTIVATION

Put it in your mind first and then in your body.

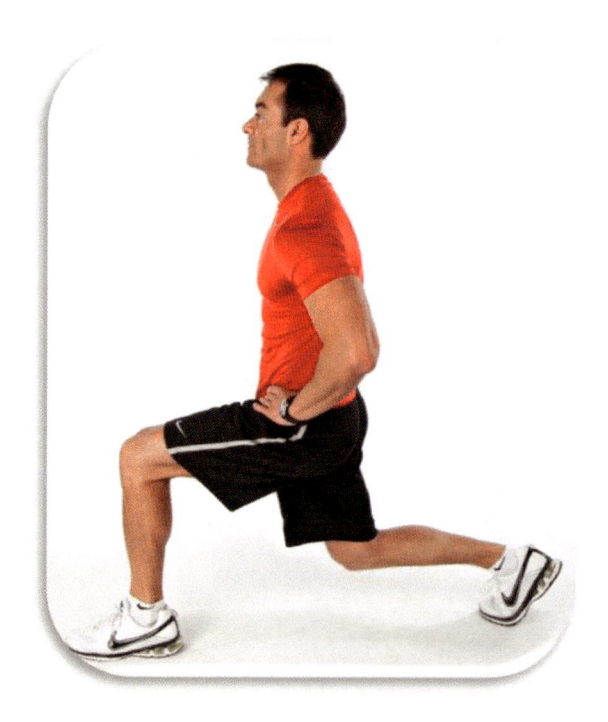

HEALTHY EATING TIP

Do not snack out of the bag; serve yourself one portion and put the rest away.

DAY 26

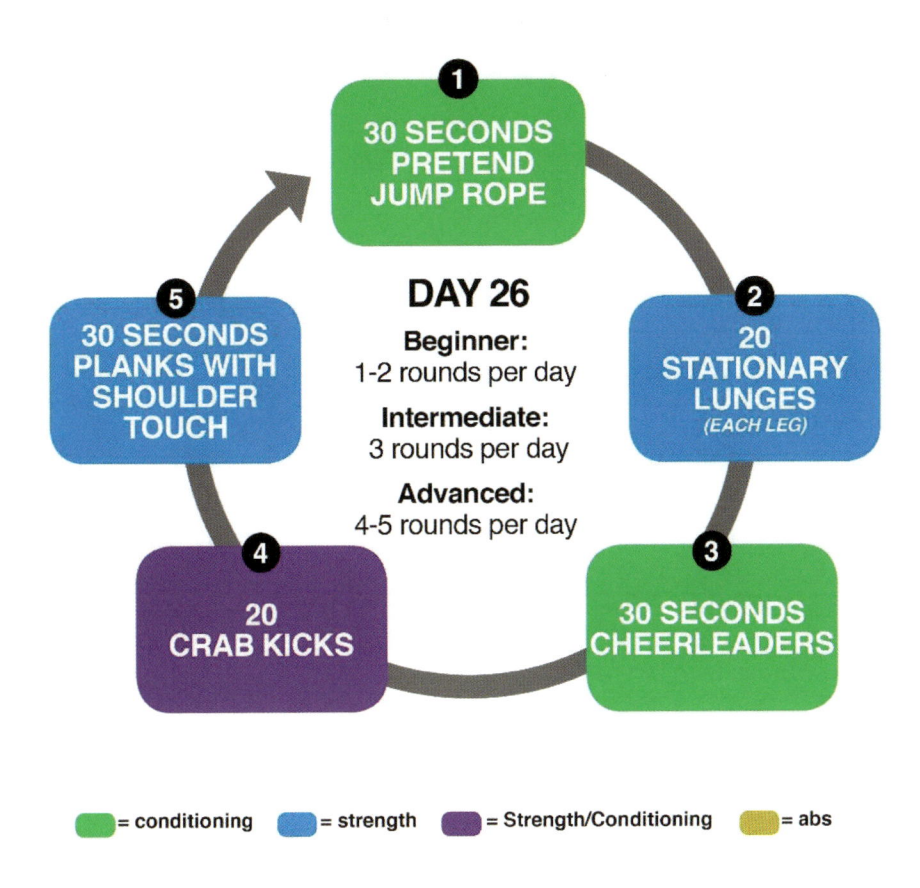

Beginner: 1-2 rounds per day

Intermediate: 3 rounds per day

Advanced: 4-5 rounds per day

1. 30 SECONDS PRETEND JUMP ROPE
2. 20 STATIONARY LUNGES (EACH LEG)
3. 30 SECONDS CHEERLEADERS
4. 20 CRAB KICKS
5. 30 SECONDS PLANKS WITH SHOULDER TOUCH

= conditioning   = strength   = Strength/Conditioning   = abs

Warm up prior to workout http://bit.ly/10YPaIU

Bonus Video-Tutorial Day 26 http://bit.ly/19fcWGM

31 DAYS OF FAT BURNING WORKOUTS

DAY 27

MOTIVATION

Workout = Endorphins = Happiness

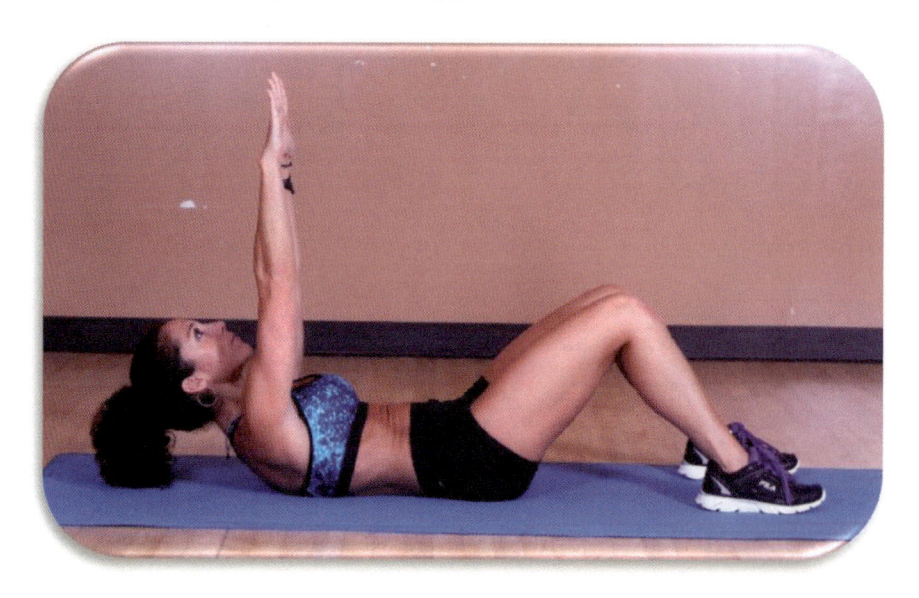

HEALTHY EATING TIP

To kill sugar cravings, eat whole fruit instead of cakes and cookies for dessert.

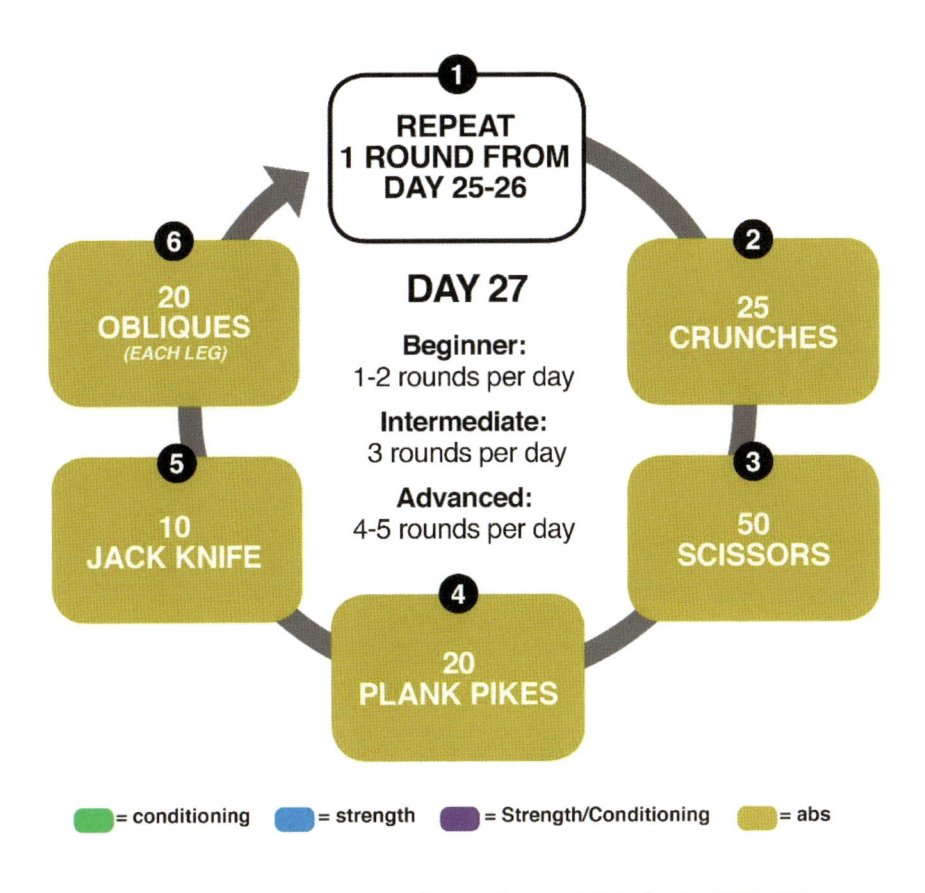

DAY 27

Beginner: 1-2 rounds per day

Intermediate: 3 rounds per day

Advanced: 4-5 rounds per day

1. REPEAT 1 ROUND FROM DAY 25-26
2. 25 CRUNCHES
3. 50 SCISSORS
4. 20 PLANK PIKES
5. 10 JACK KNIFE
6. 20 OBLIQUES (EACH LEG)

= conditioning   = strength   = Strength/Conditioning   = abs

Warm up prior to workout http://bit.ly/10YPaIU

Bonus Video-Tutorial Day 27 http://bit.ly/19fd0pW

31 DAYS OF FAT BURNING WORKOUTS

DAY 28

Beginner: 1-2 rounds per day

Intermediate: 3 rounds per day

Advanced: 4-5 rounds per day

1. 20 SQUAT KICKS
2. 30 SECONDS HALF BURPEES
3. 20 LOW CALF RAISES
4. 30 SECONDS SKATERS
5. 6-10 PUSH UPS WITH ARM LIFTS

= conditioning　　= strength　　= Strength/Conditioning　　= abs

Warm up prior to workout http://bit.ly/10YPaIU

Bonus Video-Tutorial Day 28 http://bit.ly/10JbVE0

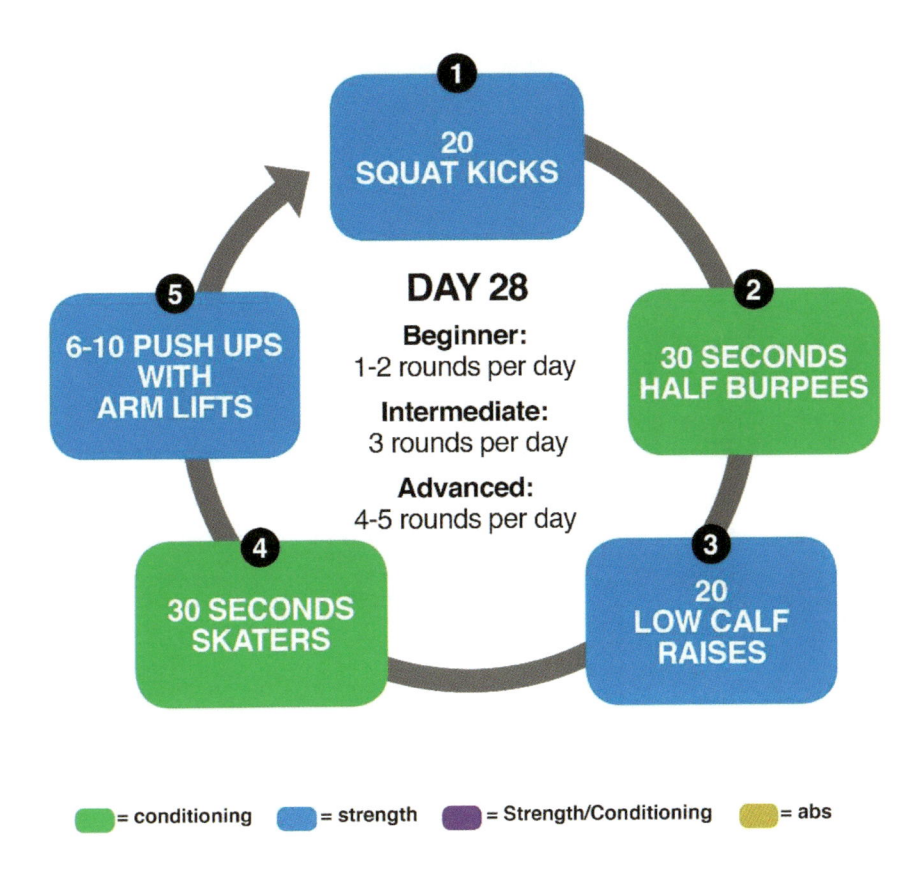

31 DAYS OF FAT BURNING WORKOUTS

DAY 29

MOTIVATION

Your body is a masterpiece, take care of it.

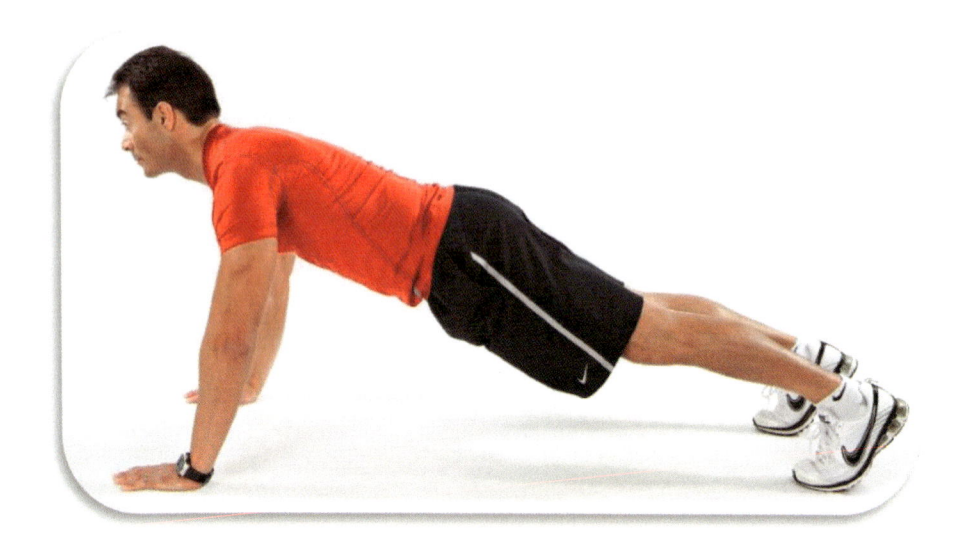

HEALTHY EATING TIP

Remove one half of the bread from your sandwich to reduce calorie intake.

31 DAYS OF FAT BURNING WORKOUTS

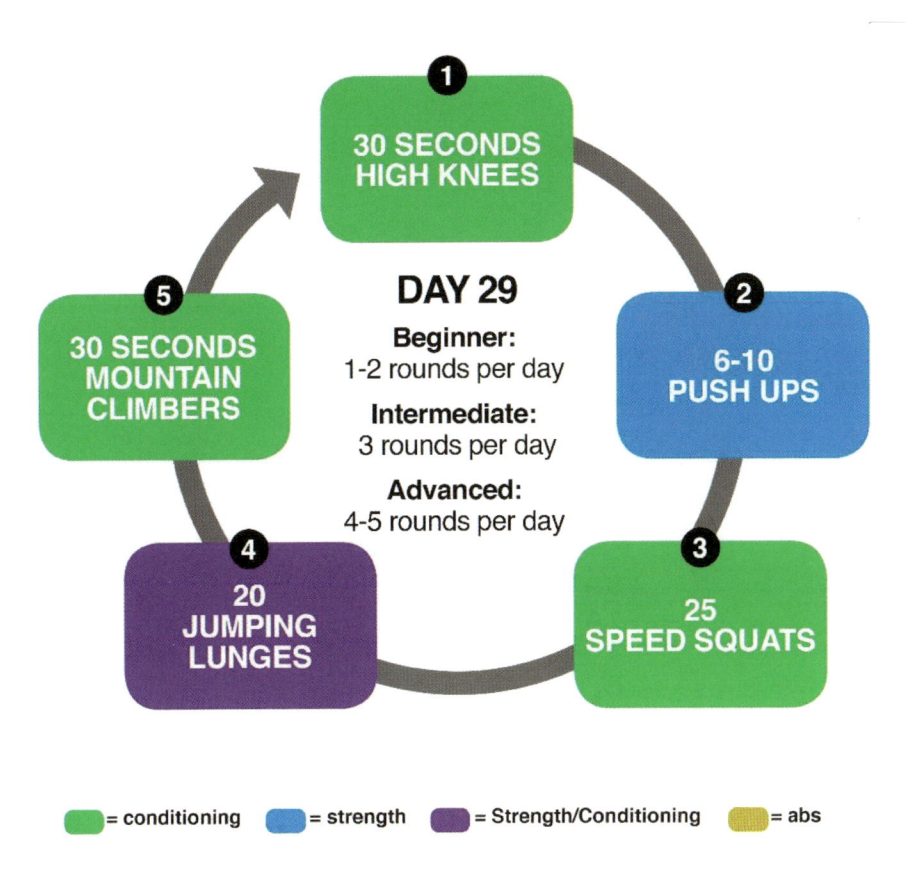

DAY 29

Beginner: 1-2 rounds per day
Intermediate: 3 rounds per day
Advanced: 4-5 rounds per day

1. 30 SECONDS HIGH KNEES
2. 6-10 PUSH UPS
3. 25 SPEED SQUATS
4. 20 JUMPING LUNGES
5. 30 SECONDS MOUNTAIN CLIMBERS

■ = conditioning ■ = strength ■ = Strength/Conditioning ■ = abs

Warm up prior to workout http://bit.ly/10YPaIU

Bonus Video-Tutorial Day 29 http://bit.ly/15t0mkF

- 77 -

31 DAYS OF FAT BURNING WORKOUTS

DAY 30

MOTIVATION

Don't diet, create a healthy lifestyle.

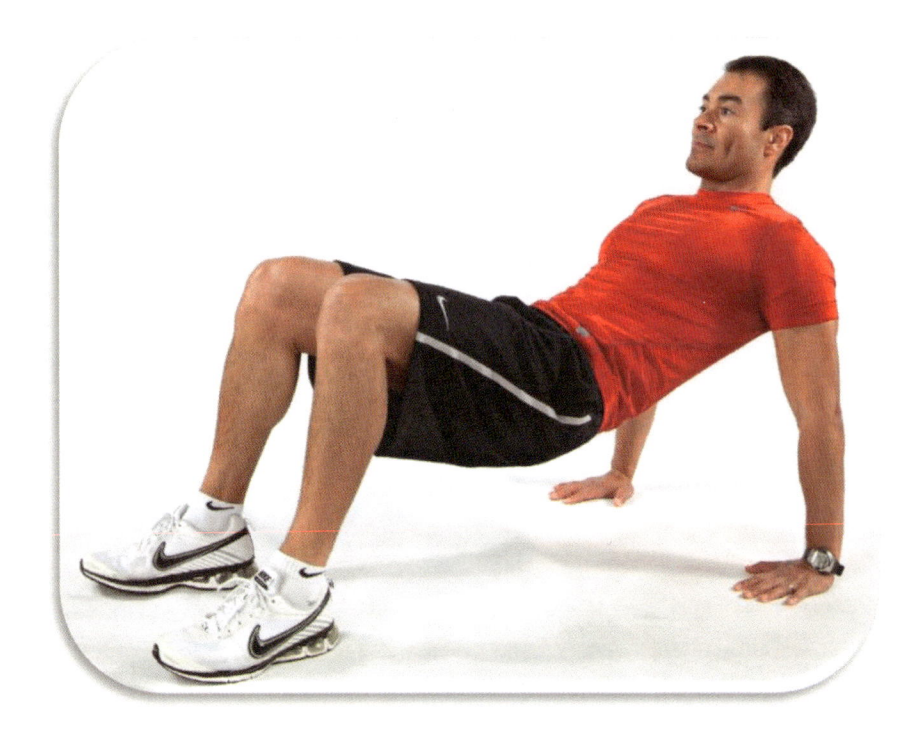

HEALTHY EATING TIP

Replace your side of french fries with a healthy salad or a bowl of low-fat soup.

DAY 30

MOTIVATION

Don't diet, create a healthy lifestyle.

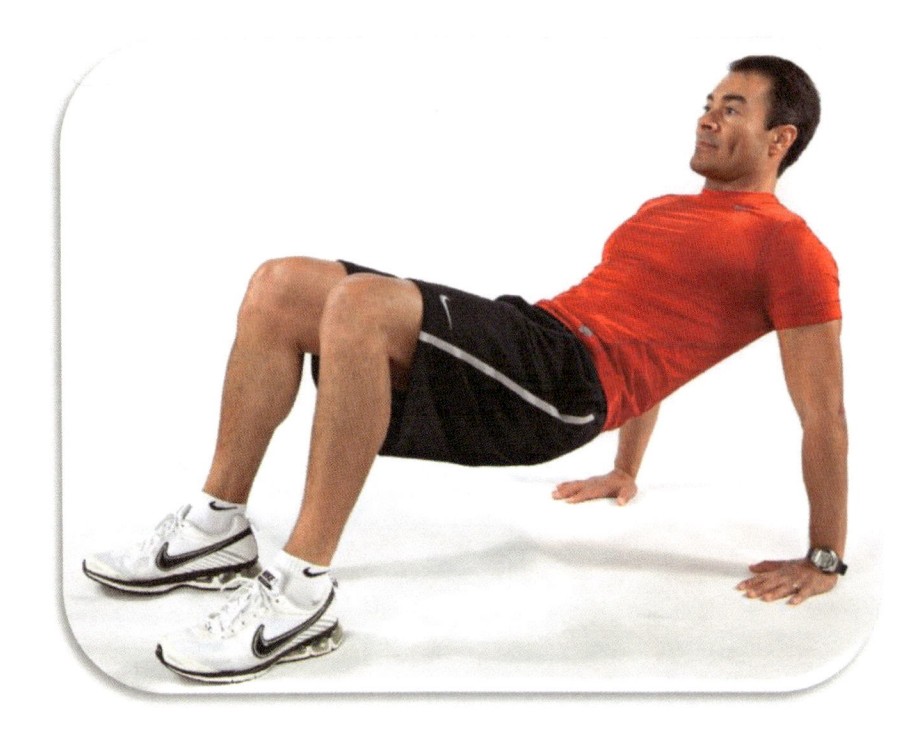

HEALTHY EATING TIP

Replace your side of french fries with a healthy salad or a bowl of low-fat soup.

31 DAYS OF FAT BURNING WORKOUTS

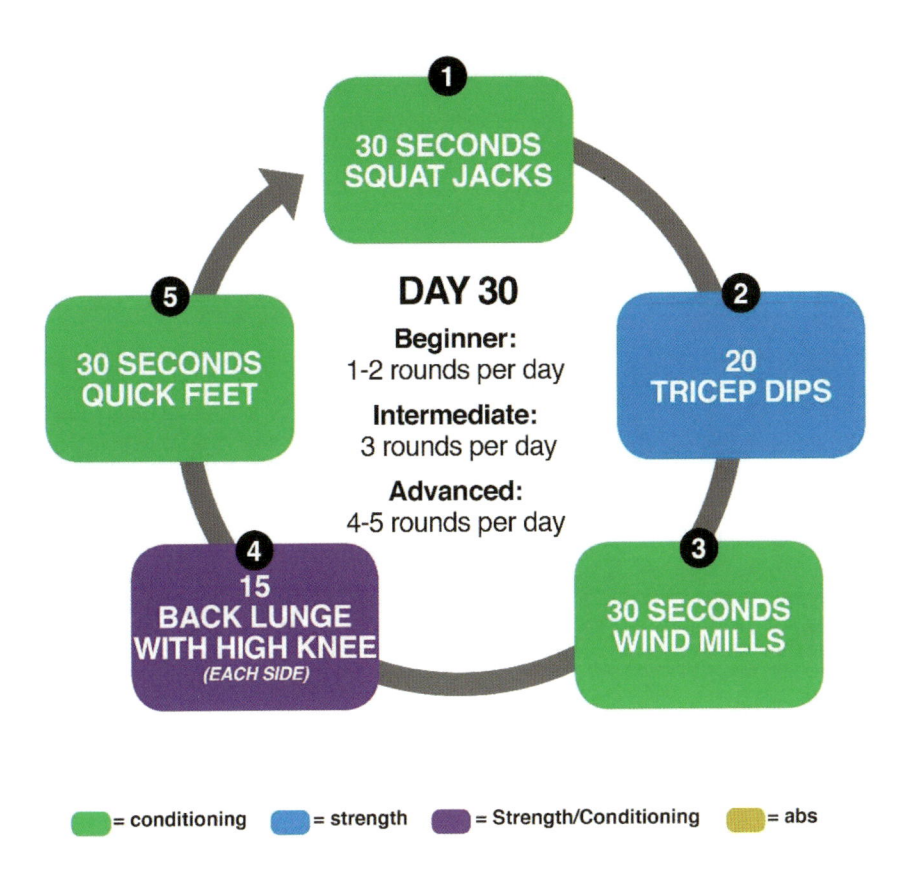

DAY 30

1. 30 SECONDS SQUAT JACKS
2. 20 TRICEP DIPS
3. 30 SECONDS WIND MILLS
4. 15 BACK LUNGE WITH HIGH KNEE (EACH SIDE)
5. 30 SECONDS QUICK FEET

Beginner: 1-2 rounds per day

Intermediate: 3 rounds per day

Advanced: 4-5 rounds per day

- = conditioning
- = strength
- = Strength/Conditioning
- = abs

Warm up prior to workout http://bit.ly/10YPaIU

Bonus Video-Tutorial Day 30 http://bit.ly/11fhNBu

31 DAYS OF FAT BURNING WORKOUTS

DAY 31

MOTIVATION

Age is not related to exercise.

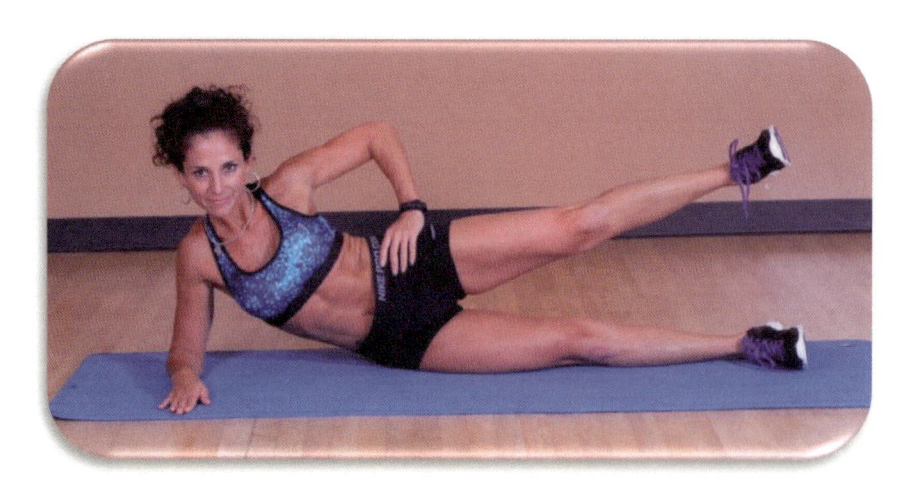

HEALTHY EATING TIP

Replace larger tortillas, pitas or slices of sandwich bread with smaller versions (10" tortillas replaced with 6" tortillas).

31 DAYS OF FAT BURNING WORKOUTS

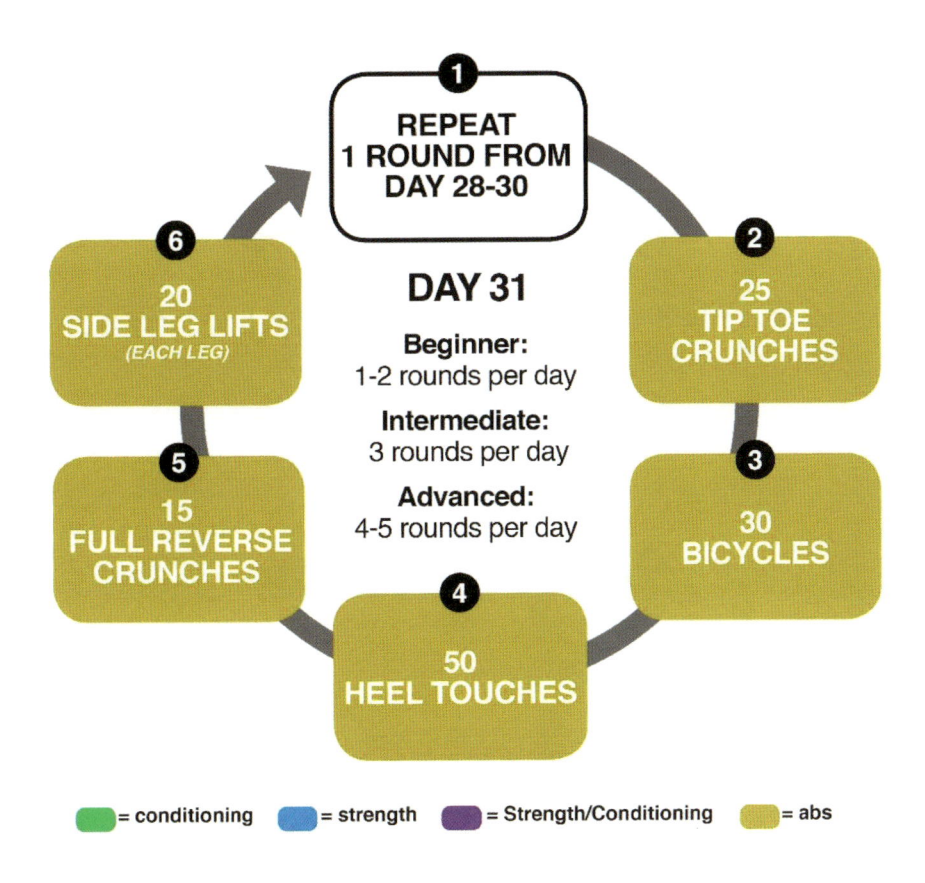

DAY 31

1. REPEAT 1 ROUND FROM DAY 28-30
2. 25 TIP TOE CRUNCHES
3. 30 BICYCLES
4. 50 HEEL TOUCHES
5. 15 FULL REVERSE CRUNCHES
6. 20 SIDE LEG LIFTS (EACH LEG)

Beginner: 1-2 rounds per day

Intermediate: 3 rounds per day

Advanced: 4-5 rounds per day

■ = conditioning   ■ = strength   ■ = Strength/Conditioning   ■ = abs

Warm up prior to workout http://bit.ly/10YPaIU

Bonus Video-Tutorial Day 31 http://bit.ly/11kmY6j

ABOUT THE AUTHOR

I am a fitness professional who launched Spin-Fit™, the first flying disc with exercises, to help fight childhood obesity. I am also an author, columnist, fitness consultant, inventor, fitness actor/model, video producer, and entrepreneur at the Trainer, LLC.

The Trainer, LLC is a company that provides health & fitness products and services in Atlanta, Georgia. The Trainer, LLC is also the manufacturer and distributor of Spin-Fit™. Our goal is to encourage and motivate children and adults to develop their own passion for sports and fitness and to develop healthy lifestyles.

For more information, please visit www.spin-fit.com.

FITNESS CREDENTIALS

- Certified Personal Trainer by the American College of Sports Medicine (ACSM)
- Certified Fitness Nutrition Coach by the National Exercise & Sports Trainers Association (NESTA)
- Certified Spinning Instructor by Mad Dogg Athletics (MDA), and Keiser
- Certified Youth Soccer Trainer/Coach by the United States Soccer Federation (USSF)

TV & FILM APPEARANCES

- USA - "Necessary Roughness" season 3 – episode 3 as Boot Camp Instructor – Sergeant Bill
- Univision 34 Atlanta – Fitness contributor since 2011

31 DAYS OF FAT BURNING WORKOUTS

- GPB "Georgia Weighs In Summit on Childhood Obesity" participating in fitness assessments
- GPB – Georgia Traveler "Exhale Spa/Gym" as Personal Trainer
- CNN "Playing sports at an early age" Interviewed by Gloria Rodriguez-Mulloy
- Azteca America Atlanta TV – Leading group exercise class with weights
- Soccer Documentary "Latino and American Soccer Leagues in Atlanta" by Will Edmonds - soccer player contributor

Connect with Trainer Marcelo on Facebook
http://on.fb.me/17EfkVZ

Made in the USA
Lexington, KY
20 August 2014